The Social and Interpersonal Origins of Depression Today

Originally published as a special issue of *Psychoanalytic Psychotherapy*, this collection was timed to coincide with the publication of the new NICE guideline for the treatment of depression, which will shape the context of NHS talking therapy services for the next decade.

In 2005, Professor Lord Layard demonstrated for the first time that mental health should matter to the UK Treasury. Layard showed that the cost of untreated depression was huge due to welfare spending on invalidity benefits, and that this was a social problem rising across the OECD, but more so in the UK. NICE had already published a clinical guideline recommending several talking therapies that were cost-effective. Why could no one still get them? In 2007, under New Labour, the world's first universal free-at-the-point-of-need service was launched to remedy this: IAPT *Improving Access to Psychological Therapies*.

Thus began a race against depression, predicted by the World Health Organisation to become the leading cause of disability worldwide by 2020. But on the eve of NICE's new guideline for depression, due in 2021, it is now clear that across large parts of the UK we are set to lose this race. Badly. Why? What went wrong? Clarke, Cundy and Yakeley have brought together a group of researchers and experts in this collection who address some of the fundamental flaws in the policy design for IAPT.

By drawing attention to neglected social and interpersonal origins of depression, pointing us towards more effective approaches, and seeking to pinpoint some of the gaps in thinking during IAPT's first decade, this book offers alternative answers to what still remains Britain's biggest social problem.

Jeremy Clarke CBE FBACP is Clinical Director at Albany Trust and a Research Associate at the Centre for Philosophy of Natural and Social Sciences, London School of Economics & at the Centre for Humanities Engaging Science and Society, Durham University. He is an Expert Member, NICE Depression guidelines (2009 & 2021 forthcoming), and former National Adviser, Improving Access to Psychological Therapies (2008–2013).

Paul Cundy is a Consultant Adult Psychotherapist and a Psychodynamic Psychotherapy Lead at North East London NHS Foundation Trust, UK. He is an Associate Fellow of the British Psychological Society, Leicester, UK and Assistant Editor of *Psychoanalytic Psychotherapy.*

Jessica Yakeley is a Consultant Psychiatrist in Forensic Psychotherapy, Director of the Portman Clinic, and Director of Medical Education at the Tavistock and Portman NHS Foundation Trust, London, UK. She is a fellow of the British Psychoanalytical Society, London, UK and Editor of *Psychoanalytic Psychotherapy.*

The Social and Interpersonal Origins of Depression Today

Edited by
Jeremy Clarke, Paul Cundy and Jessica Yakeley

Routledge
Taylor & Francis Group
LONDON AND NEW YORK

First published 2020
by Routledge
2 Park Square, Milton Park, Abingdon, Oxon, OX14 4RN

and by Routledge
52 Vanderbilt Avenue, New York, NY 10017

Routledge is an imprint of the Taylor & Francis Group, an informa business

British Library Cataloguing-in-Publication Data
A catalogue record for this book is available from the British Library

ISBN13: 978-0-367-45898-0

Typeset in Times New Roman
by codeMantra

Publisher's Note
The publisher accepts responsibility for any inconsistencies that may have arisen during the conversion of this book from journal articles to book chapters, namely the inclusion of journal terminology.

Contents

Citation Information

The chapters in this book were originally published in the *Psychoanalytic Psychotherapy*, volume 32, issue 02 (June 2018). When citing this material, please use the original page numbering for each article, as follows:

Guest editorial

Jeremy Clarke
Psychoanalytic Psychotherapy, volume 32, issue 02 (June 2018) pp. 95–101

Chapter 1

Epistemological flaws in NICE review methodology and its impact on recommendations for psychodynamic psychotherapies for complex and persistent depression
Susan McPherson, Felicitas Rost, Joel Town & Allan Abbass
Psychoanalytic Psychotherapy, volume 32, issue 02 (June 2018) pp. 102–121

Chapter 2

The interpersonal structure of depression
Matthew Ratcliffe
Psychoanalytic Psychotherapy, volume 32, issue 02 (June 2018) pp. 122–139

Chapter 3

The active ingredients of dynamic interpersonal therapy (DIT): an exploration of clients' experiences
Venetia Leonidaki, Alessandra Lemma & Imogen Hobbis
Psychoanalytic Psychotherapy, volume 32, issue 02 (June 2018) pp. 140–156

Chapter 4

The process of change in ethnic minority males undergoing psychodynamic psychotherapy: a detailed comparison of two cases
Tohar Dolev, Sigal Zilcha-Mano, Harold Chui, Marna S. Barrett, Kevin S. McCarthy & Jacques P. Barber
Psychoanalytic Psychotherapy, volume 32, issue 02 (June 2018) pp. 157–180

Chapter 5
The secret sorrows of men: impact of Dynamic Interpersonal Therapy on 'masculine depression'
Joanna S. Dognin & Cory K. Chen
Psychoanalytic Psychotherapy, volume 32, issue 02 (June 2018) pp. 181–196

Chapter 6
'Post-natal' depression in fathers, or Early Fatherhood Depression
Sameer P. Sarkar
Psychoanalytic Psychotherapy, volume 32, issue 02 (June 2018) pp. 197–216

Chapter 7
Influence of childhood trauma on depression in the INDDEP study
Anna Lea Docter, Almut Zeeck, Jörn von Wietersheim & Heinz Weiss
Psychoanalytic Psychotherapy, volume 32, issue 02 (June 2018) pp. 217–234

Contributors

Allan Abbass is a Professor at Faculty of Medicine, Centre for Emotions and Health, Dalhousie University, Halifax, Canada.

Jacques P. Barber is Professor and Dean at the Gordon F. Derner School of Psychology, Adelphi University, Garden City, NY, USA.

Marna S. Barrett is an Adjunct Associate Professor at Department of Psychiatry, University of Pennsylvania, Philadelphia, USA.

Jeremy Clarke CBE FBACP is Clinical Director at Albany Trust and a Research Associate at the Centre for Philosophy of Natural and Social Sciences, London School of Economics & at the Centre for Humanities Engaging Science and Society, Durham University. He is an Expert Member, NICE Depression guidelines (2009 & 2021 forthcoming), and former National Adviser, Improving Access to Psychological Therapies (2008–2013).

Cory K. Chen is Director of the Psychotherapy Research and Development Program at the VA New York Harbor Healthcare System and an Associate Professor at Department of Psychiatry, New York University School of Medicine, USA.

Harold Chui is a Professor at Department of Educational Psychology, The Chinese University of Hong Kong, Shatin, Hong Kong.

Paul Cundy is a Consultant Adult Psychotherapist and a Psychodynamic Psychotherapy Lead at North East London NHS Foundation Trust, UK. He is an Associate Fellow of the British Psychological Society, Leicester, UK and Assistant Editor of *Psychoanalytic Psychotherapy*.

Anna Lea Docter is a Medical Doctor at Department for Psychiatry, Psychosomatic Medicine and Psychotherapy, University Medical Center, Frankfurt am Main, Germany. She is a Research Associate and Medical Doctor at Sigmund Freud Institut, Frankfurt am Main, Germany.

Joanna S. Dognin is an Assistant Professor at Department of Psychiatry, New York University School of Medicine, USA.

Tohar Dolev is a Doctoral Candidate at Department of Psychology, University of Haifa, Israel.

Imogen Hobbis is a Clinical Psychologist and a Clinical Senior Lecturer in Clinical Psychology at the University of East Anglia.

Alessandra Lemma is a Visiting Professor in the Psychoanalysis Unit at UCL and a Consultant Clinical Psychologist, Anna Freud National Centre.

Venetia Leonidaki is a Consultant Clinical Psychologist at Central and North West London Foundation Trust, an Accredited Psychotherapist (BABCP, BCP) and a Visiting Lecturer.

Kevin S. McCarthy is an Associate Professor at Department of Psychology, Chestnut Hill College, Philadelphia, USA.

Susan McPherson is a Senior Lecturer at School of Health and Social Care, University of Essex, Colchester, UK.

Matthew Ratcliffe is Professor of Philosophy at the University of York, UK. Most of his recent work addresses issues in phenomenology, philosophy of mind, and philosophy of psychiatry. He is author of *Rethinking Commonsense Psychology: A Critique of Folk Psychology, Theory of Mind and Simulation* (Palgrave, 2007), *Feelings of Being: Phenomenology, Psychiatry and the Sense of Reality* (Oxford University Press, 2008), *Experiences of Depression: A Study in Phenomenology* (Oxford University Press, 2015), and *Real Hallucinations: Psychiatric Illness, Intentionality, and the Interpersonal World* (MIT Press, 2017).

Felicitas Rost is a Research Lead at Portman Clinic, Tavistock and Portman NHS Foundation Trust, London, UK.

Sameer P. Sarkar Sameer P. Sarkar is a Consultant in Psychiatry and Forensic Psychiatry with the Ministry of Defence. He is based in Aldershot Centre for Health, Hampshire, as the clinical lead for Department of Community Mental Health, part of the Joint Medical Group.

Joel Town is an Assistant Professor at Faculty of Medicine, Department of Psychiatry, Dalhousie University, Halifax, Canada.

Heinz Weiss is a Head of at the Department of Psychosomatic Medicine of the Robert-Bosch-Krankenhaus, Stuttgart, Germany.

Jörn von Wietersheim is a Professor at Department for Psychosomatic Medicine and Psychotherapy, Medical University Medical Center, Ulm, Germany.

Jessica Yakeley is a Consultant Psychiatrist in Forensic Psychotherapy, Director of the Portman Clinic, and Director of Medical Education at the Tavistock and Portman NHS Foundation Trust, London, UK. She is a fellow of the British Psychoanalytical Society, London, UK and Editor of *Psychoanalytic Psychotherapy.*

Almut Zeeck is a Professor at Department for Psychosomatic Medicine and Psychotherapy, University Medical Center, Freiburg, Germany.

Sigal Zilcha-Mano is an Associate Professor at Department of Psychology, University of Haifa, Israel.

Introduction

Jeremy Clarke

The day of the bog-standard comprehensive is over (Alistair Campbell, 2001)

This special issue on depression is timed to coincide with a new National Institute for Health and Care Excellence (NICE) guideline (forthcoming). It will be NICE's 3rd depression guideline, the first in 2004, the second in 2009. Improving Access to Psychological Therapies (IAPT)'s ubiquitous stepped care model, which has gained international recognition for its 'world-leading results' (Stevens, 2017), derives from NICE's depression guidelines (NICE, 2009). So, it is safe to say this latest iteration will shape the context for NHS-funded talking therapy services for the next decade.

What was the impact of NICE's first two guidelines? Thanks to two independent National Audits (Royal College of Psychiatrists, 2011, 2013), a wealth of outcomes data from IAPT itself (NHS Digital, 2015–16, 2016–17), the recent Psychiatric Morbidity Survey (McManus, Bebbington, Jenkins, & Brugha, 2016), and detailed prescribing data for anti-depressants (HSCIC, 2016), we are in a good position to track NICE's impact over the last 10 years.

However, the story can only be understood fully against the context of a radical attempt to create a comprehensive 'universal access' talking therapies NHS service, free-at-the-point-of-need to all: 'You are deprived if you cannot enjoy your life. And the most common cause of deprivation is not poverty or unemployment but mental illness' (Clark, Fleche, Layard, Powdthavee, & Ward, 2018). Professor Lord Richard Layard's (2005) flawed but brilliantly original analysis for the Prime Minister's Strategy Unit argued that depression causes the UK's single greatest disease burden not only due to its prevalence but also its indirect welfare costs. In other words, invalidity due to chronic depression was to blame for rapidly rising welfare spending occurring across the member countries of the Organisation for Economic Co-operation and Development (OECD), but especially so in the UK (Organisation for Economic Co-operation & Development, 2012). Layard's solution was simple. NICE had identified cognitive behavioural therapy (CBT) as the most cost-effective treatment for common mental illness, Q.E.D. create a comprehensive Improving Access to CBT service, 'which will pay for itself'. In 2007, Layard and I met with Treasury officials at Number 10 Downing Street.[1] We secured a business case for investing in talking *therapies* to the tune of £300 million in its first three years. IAPT went on to get £400 million under the Coalition; and then a further £600 million from George Osborne[2]'s spending review.

This unprecedented level of investment has shaped the nature and evolution of adult National Health Service (NHS) talking therapy services for the foreseeable future, and is set to do likewise for children and young people. Although there was an accidental element to finding myself a National Adviser to IAPT, and an apologist in public, at least, for how we built its infrastructure, it was also as a result of a clear-eyed plan with colleagues (Lemma & Allen, 2010) to shore up the vulnerable position of psychoanalytic psychotherapy in the NHS as we entered a prolonged period of austerity. When the Royal College of Psychiatrists appointed me to lead the 2nd independent National Audit of NHS psychotherapy services (2013), I also had a good opportunity to assess IAPT's progress towards a comprehensive service, and the extent to which we were delivering on the promises we made to Government. So, as well as describing what we know about the impact of NICE and IAPT to date, I want to use the opportunity of this editorial to offer brief personal reflections on what I think will be the challenges facing us over the next decade, and which I hope the papers in this special edition bring into view.

At around the same time that Phil Richardson and his colleagues embarked upon the Tavistock Adult Depression Study (Fonagy et al., 2015), another study was reported in the British Medical Journal that illustrated how short a step it is from the most 'sublime', flawlessly designed randomized controlled trial (RCT), to the most 'ridiculous', yet scientifically 'rigorous' findings for a treatment effect (Leibovici, 2001). The study reported an intervention with a patient sample of 3393 patients who were the total number of patients with sepsis-related blood infection in one hospital setting over a period of 6 years. They were randomized into two parallel groups who were matched on risk factors for mortality. The design was 'double blind plus', as neither patients nor staff knew which group the patients were allocated to, and didn't even know the trial was happening because it took place retro-actively. The intervention was remote, retro-active *praying* for the treatment group, none for the control group, and the effects measured were: the number of deaths in hospital, length of stay in hospital from the day of the first positive blood culture to discharge or death and duration of fever. Patients were defined as having fever on a specific day if one of three temperature measurements taken on that day showed a temperature of >37.5 °C. Results were that remote, retroactive intercessory prayer was associated with a shorter stay in hospital and a shorter duration of fever in patients with a bloodstream infection. Mortality was lower in the intervention group, but the difference between the groups was not significant. A larger study might have shown a significant reduction in mortality.

I use this example to make a serious point about NICE's flawed approach to evaluating evidence, which McPherson et al.'s sustained critique in this issue of NICE's depression guideline (on which I was an expert committee member) develops further. Evidence from RCTs, we are told, is the only kind of evidence that can *clinch* a causal claim that this treatment X worked better than that treatment Y. The argument is that other kinds of evidence, for example, observational studies following a cohort of people, such as those undertaken by Brown and Harris (1978) on a group of women with depression can, at best, as Nancy Cartwright (2011) puts it only *vouch for* a causal claim – in this case, that a major interpersonal loss can precipitate depression, and that a trusted source of emotional support can help mitigate it.

The criticisms made against Brown and Harris are typical of the concerns about bias, error and supposed rigour that dominate NICE's approach to evaluation, viz: '(i) the methods of selecting patients are open to contamination by the views of the investigators; (ii) the procedure for eliciting life events is unvalidated; (iii) the assessment of the severity of life events is based almost entirely upon the subjective judgements of a handful of investigators; (iv) the methods of analysing data appear to be selective and ambiguous; and (v) important conclusions often seem to be inconsistent with the findings' (Shapiro, 1979). But as Cartwright and Deaton (2016) have shown, these criticisms apply equally to assumptions intrinsic to RCTs, which neither randomization, nor blinding, nor fidelity of intervention, nor impressive effect sizes, as the Leibovici study *perfectly* illustrates, can add up to predict our wished-for inference, 'this treatment will work for me', will be guaranteed.

If, according to advocates of RCTs, we are forced to conclude that someone praying that a patient will get better, who never sees that patient nor knows anything about them and who is praying for them in a different place and at a different time, after the fact of their illness and recovery, indeed, and who neither the patient, nor their medical team, nor anyone else at the time knew about, nevertheless was able to bring about a speedier recovery, as *proven* by an impeccable RCT, something is wrong! And if, then, these are the only building blocks thrown together in a network meta-analysis with its own additional questionable assumptions, as McPherson et al. show, we have reason for concern.

Perhaps the more trenchant criticism, however, concerns NICE's paltry lip service to the patient's subjective experience of depression. An underlying difficulty here, which Matthew Ratcliffe rightly pinpoints in his impressive article on the interpersonal structure of depression, is the a-theoretical vacuum created when psychiatry moved away from an explanatory nosology for classifying mental illness roughly from the third edition of DSM onwards. Without an adequate grounding in how people experience depression today, however, it is difficult to know what an 'evidence-based' treatment for depression is actually treating, let alone whether we can know how or why it works. Both Ratcliffe and Leonidaki and colleagues start to redress the gap using evidence from first-person accounts.

The significance of these two articles, well-founded as they are, suggests a serious conceptual error – described as 'diagnostic literalism' (Kendler, 2016) – where the reification of specific symptoms of depression as the targets for our treatment interventions, driven on by the ambition of achieving parity of esteem with anti-depressant medications, is akin to mistaking the shadows on the wall of Plato's allegorical cave for the real thing itself. Notwithstanding the hype greeting the network meta-analysis of anti-depressants published in the Lancet by Cipriani et al. (2018), the differences between the drug treatment and placebo in more recent placebo-controlled trials were still found to be small. Similarly, effects of CBT as a treatment for depression have also been found to be falling in more recent RCTs (Johnsen & Friborg, 2015). The optimistic view may be that so-called placebo effects are proving potent in their own right (Kirsch, Wampold, & Kelley, 2016). But if Ratcliffe is right about the centrality of interpersonal experience in depression, and I think he is, then unless they start to make more explicit use of this in the therapeutic relationship, for example, neither anti-depressants nor CBT may have much of a future. The challenge for contemporary dynamic therapies, such as Dynamic Interpersonal Therapy, which already use a relational focus to elicit interpersonal aspects of depression, as Leonidaki et al. demonstrate, is now to begin to explore causal relationships and interactions between underlying structures, manifest symptoms, and the complex relational and technical factors that lead to change. Identifying patients' explanations for DIT's efficacy has given us some useful facts on the ground.

The next three articles introduce a pressing question since the pioneering work of Brown and Harris with women: What does the interpersonal structure of depression look like for men? The reason this is urgent is because it relates to how depression for men can impact on their capacity to work and is driving increased suicides. Every week in the UK 84 men die by suicide. A toxic combination of unemployment and depression has impacted especially on men aged 45–64 since the financial crash (Barr et al., 2012); for men under 45 suicide is the biggest killer. Amongst social security (Employment and Support Allowance) claimants, rates of self-harm and chronic depression are at alarming levels (McManus et al., 2016).

Dolev and colleagues report an evidence-based case study that compares two ethnic minority males undertaking brief dynamic therapy with contrasting outcomes. This article was the winning entry in our case study prize. It elegantly shows how case studies can tease out knowledge of what works (or not) for whom by shedding light on a key process. In the two reported cases, when the therapist took a risk but caused a rupture, which she then had to work to repair, improvement followed. The unimproved client appeared to find therapy supportive but remained at a distance. Another recent study corroborates this finding (Werbart, von Below, Engqvist, & Lind, 2018). Understanding what *doesn't* work for whom is as much a priority as what does. Unimproved cases probably account for 80–90% of the total IAPT caseload, most of whom have received CBT, though not by their own choice (Tasca, Town, Abbass, & Clarke, in press).

Dognin and Chen describe the application of DIT in the context of a New York clinic for USA military veterans. They highlight the urgent need for such help in America when 20 veterans a day are reportedly committing suicide, almost twice the average annual figure for the total number of all suicides in the UK (Appleby et al., 2017). The value of Dognin and Chen's work with a particular group of men for whom we can probably add trauma into the case mix, alongside risk of self-harm and depression, is their way of applying DIT to understand what we could call – *the social origins of hegemonic masculinity* and its role in the pathology of what is termed here *masculine depression*. Sarkar is also concerned with how an insecure gender identity is implicated in depression in men. His review of the literature shows both how post-natal depression can develop in some men as well as how it often goes unidentified. The targets for the 20 new perinatal services set up with £40 million funding by NHS England, for example, refer solely to access for 9000 more women in 2018/19. The exemplar case Sarkar describes illuminates a complex process of internalized stigma, emotional conflict and inter-generational transmission of pathogenic identifications. Common to all three articles that explore the interpersonal structure of depression in men is a relational approach that enables experience of what Dognin and Chen identify as 'caring masculinity' (Green, Emslie, O'Neill, Hunt, & Walker, 2010). The role model for this in the UK, as NHS provision for veterans has expanded, is Prince Harry.

The final article empirically establishes the causal impact of childhood trauma on depressive illness. The careful, nuanced picture that we are presented with by Docter and colleagues, stands in contrast to the somewhat crude version of stepped care – two sizes fit all – that IAPT adopted from NICE.

Our present dilemma, here, is that RCTs are held to be the 'gold standard' and the only currency NICE committees will accept. NICE guidelines, likewise, are the basis on which commissioning decisions are made. If psychoanalytic psychotherapy cannot gain and hold on to a place as a recommended treatment in NICE guidelines, therefore, we are effectively finished as a discipline in NHS funded mental health services. McPherson et al. demonstrate this is a marathon not a sprint.

There are three clear challenges, in my view, that face our own discipline over the next decade. First, we must recognize, as with the radical policy shift that took place in education with the introduction of comprehensive schools to provide equal opportunities for all, that in order to engage productively with the NICE-IAPT axis of universal mental healthcare we must embrace short-term dynamic therapy. Whatever the collateral damage done by IAPT's relentless focus on access targets (we have been drawing attention to staff burnout, for example) (New Savoy Partnership/British Psychological Society, 2018), the fact that almost all patients can now be guaranteed access to talking therapies within 6 weeks is an undeniably huge achievement. Second, however, if the goal of evidence-based practice is to offer equity of access to 'gold standard' therapies, what I would call 'evidence-best practice', and with the policy aim of reducing the burden of disease, the lessons from IAPT are clear. All the indicators have moved in the wrong direction. As I hope this collection of articles demonstrates, until and unless our philosophy of science becomes more sophisticated in relation to the context for particular patients (e.g. men) and the underlying mechanisms of change (e.g. something other than remote, retrospective inter-cessionary prayer!), then our service models will largely end up delivering 'bog-standard' outcomes.

Finally, I began this journey in league with Lord Layard with a promise to bring the benefit of talking therapies to people on social security as an entitlement the welfare state should offer to all. But in areas of social deprivation what we see today are recovery rates for depression following treatment with CBT and/or medication that are 20% lower than in areas of relative affluence (NHS Digital, 2015–16). When one looks at the UK atlas of variation for rates of prescribing anti-depressants now (in some areas 1 in 6 adults are on long-term medication), it correlates with the map for those areas that voted for Brexit. Is this as good as it gets? No, the job is far from done.

Notes

1. The address of the British Prime Minister.
2. Chancellor of the Exchequer under Prime Minister David Cameron from 2010 to 2016.

References

Appleby, L., Kapur, N., Shaw, J., Hunt, I. M., Ibrahim, S., Gianatsi, M., … Raphael, J. (2017, October). *The national confidential inquiry into suicide and homicide by people with mental illness*. Annual Report. Manchester: University of Manchester.

Barr, B., Taylor-Robinson, D., Scott-Samuel, A., McKee, M., & Stuckler, D. (2012). Suicides associated with the 2008–10 economic recession in England: Time trend analysis. *BMJ, 345*, e5142. doi: 10.1136/bmj.e5142

Brown, G. W., & Harris, T. (1978). *Social origins of depression: A study of psychiatric disorder in women*. London: Tavistock.

Campbell, A. (2001). Retrieved from https://www.theguardian.com/education/2009/dec/08/education-policy-schools-labour

Cartwright, N. (2011). A philosopher's view of the long road from RCTs to effectiveness. *The Lancet, 377*(9775), 1400–1401.

Cartwright, N., & Deaton, A. (2016). *Understanding and misunderstanding randomized controlled trials*. Working paper. Durham: Centre for Humanities Engaging Science and Society and National Bureau of Economic Research.

Cipriani, A., Furukawa, T. A., Salanti, G., Chaimani, A., Atkinson, L. Z., Ogawa, Y., … Geddes, J. R. (2018). Comparative efficacy and acceptability of 21 antidepressant drugs for the acute treatment of adults with major depressive disorder: A systematic review and network meta-analysis. *The Lancet, 391*(10128), 1357–1366. doi:10.1016/S0140-6736(17)32802-7

Clark, A. E., Fleche, S., Layard, R., Powdthavee, N., & Ward, G. (2018). *The origins of happiness: The science of well-being over the life course*. Princeton, NJ: Princeton University Press.

Fonagy, P., Rost, F., Carlyle, J., McPherson, S., Thomas, R., Pasco Fearon, R., … Taylor, D. (2015). Pragmatic randomized controlled trial of long-term psychoanalytic psychotherapy for treatment-resistant depression: The Tavistock Adult Depression Study (TADS). *World Psychiatry, 14*(3), 312–321. doi:10.1002/wps.20267

Green, G., Emslie, C., O'Neill, D., Hunt, K., & Walker, S. (2010). Exploring the ambiguities of masculinity in accounts of emotional distress in the military among young ex-servicemen. *Social Science & Medicine, 71*(8), 1480–1488. doi:10.1016/j.socscimed.2010.07.015

HSCIC. (2016). *Prescriptions dispensed in the community: England 2005–15*. (Responsible Statistician Ian Bullard, Section head). Health and Social Care Information Centre. ISBN 978-1-78386-743-1 published 5th July, 2016.

Johnsen, T. J., & Friborg, O. (2015). The effects of cognitive behavioral therapy as an anti-depressive treatment is falling: A meta-analysis. *Psychological Bulletin, 141*, 747–768. doi:10.1037/bul0000015

Kendler, K. S. (2016). The phenomenology of major depression and the representativeness and nature of DSM criteria. *American Journal of Psychiatry, 173*, 771–780. doi:10.1176/appi.ajp.2016.15121509

Kirsch, I., Wampold, B., & Kelley, J. M. (2016). Controlling for the placebo effect in psychotherapy: Noble quest or tilting at windmills? *Psychology of Consciousness: Theory, Research, and Practice, 3*(2), 121–131. doi:10.1037/cns0000065

Layard, R. (2005). *The depression report: A new deal for depression and anxiety*. Retrieved from http://cep.lse.ac.uk/pubs/download/special/depressionreport.pdf

Leibovici, L. (2001). Effects of remote, retroactive intercessory prayer on outcomes in patients with bloodstream infection: Randomised controlled trial. *BMJ, 323*, 1450–1451.

Lemma, A., & Allen, M. (2010). Editorial. *Psychoanalytic Psychotherapy, 24*(1), 1–2. doi:10.1080/02668731003589388

McManus, S., Bebbington, P., Jenkins, R., & Brugha, T. (2016). *Mental health and wellbeing in England: Adult psychiatric morbidity survey 2014*. Leeds: NHS Digital.

New Savoy Partnership/British Psychological Society. (2018). Retrieved from https://www.bps.org.uk/news-and-policy/survey-mental-health-workforce-finds-many-services-compromised-staff-vacancies

NHS Digital. (2015–16, October 18). *Psychological therapies: Annual report on the use of IAPT services in England*. Leeds: NHS Digital. Retrieved from https://digital.nhs.uk/catalogue/PUB22110

NHS Digital. (2016–17, November 30). *Psychological therapies: Annual report on the use of IAPT services in England*. Leeds: NHS Digital. Retrieved from https://digital.nhs.uk/catalogue/PUB30157

NICE. (2009). *Clinical Guideline 90 Depression in Adults*. London: BPS & Royal College Psychiatrists.

NICE. (forthcoming). *Depression in Adults: Treatment and management*. London: National Guideline Alliance, hosted by the Royal College of Obstetricians and Gynaecologists.

Organisation for Economic Co-operation and Development. (2012). *Mental Health and Work: United Kingdom*. Paris: OECD. doi:10.1787/9789264204997-en

Royal College of Psychiatrists. (2011). *National Audit of Psychological Therapies for Anxiety and Depression*. National Report.

Royal College of Psychiatrists. (2013). *Report of the Second Round of the National Audit of Psychological Therapies (NAPT) 2013*. London: Healthcare Quality Improvement Partnership.

Shapiro, M. B. (1979). The social origins of depression: By G. W. Brown and T. Harris: Its methodological philosophy. *Behaviour, Research and Therapy, 17*(6), 597–603.

Stevens, S. (2017). *NHS England oral evidence to Health Select Committee, quoting New York Times report on IAPT*. Retrieved from https://www.nytimes.com/2017/07/24/health/england-mental-health-treatment-therapy.html

Tasca, G. A., Town, J. M., Abbass, A., & Clarke, J. (in press). Will publicly funded psychotherapy in Canada be evidence-based? A review of what makes psychotherapy work and a proposal. *Journal of Canadian Psychology*. Special issue on Psychotherapy forthcoming.

Werbart, A., von Below, C., Engqvist, K., & Lind, S. (2018). 'It was like having half of the patient in therapy': Therapists of nonimproved patients looking back on their work. *Psychotherapy Research*. Advance online publication. doi:10.1080/10503307.2018.1453621

Epistemological flaws in NICE review methodology and its impact on recommendations for psychodynamic psychotherapies for complex and persistent depression

Susan McPherson, Felicitas Rost, Joel Town and Allan Abbass

The UK draft NICE guideline on depression in adults was sent out for stakeholder consultation between July and September 2017. The final guideline publication date currently remains 'to be confirmed'. This paper sets out key concerns with the methodology employed in the guideline and its impact on recommendations for psychodynamic psychotherapies for complex and persistent depression. The draft largely ignored the subjective experiences and voices of service users, carers and members of the public, using out of date limited evidence of service user and carer experiences. The guideline fails to incorporate what limited qualitative evidence it reviewed into any treatment recommendations. The Guideline Committee created its own method for categorising depression by longevity, severity and complexity. This has resulted in erroneous and unhelpful classifications of research studies under groupings which do not match clinical and service user experiences or US and European approaches, rendering analyses and conclusions unreliable. We also outline instances of incorrect classification of psychodynamic treatments (such as inclusion of non bona fide treatments or exclusion of relevant bona fide treatment studies) which enables the omission of a recommendation for psychodynamic psychotherapy for complex and persistent depression. Depression is often a long-term condition or can become so if immediate care is inadequate; yet the draft recommendations are all made on the basis of short-term outcome data (with often less than eight weeks between baseline and outcome). NICE guidelines for long-term physical conditions would treat this evidence as inadequate. Finally, the draft guideline used the Grading of Recommendations, Assessment, Development and Evaluation (GRADE) system of assessing methodological quality in such a way as to produce a systematic bias in favour of drug trials, selectively omitting trial data with long-term follow-up points and those which used non-symptom outcomes. Herein, we consider the increasingly evident limitations of the paradigm NICE works within for ensuring patient choice and equity of access to a wide range of therapies.

Background

The draft NICE guideline (2017) on depression in adults was sent out for stakeholder consultation between July and September 2017 with a planned publication date of January 2018, that has since been moved twice, first to March 2018 and currently 'to be confirmed'. This pause might be an acknowledgement of the gravity of stakeholder concerns and the relevance of the guideline to public mental health. Much new evidence has emerged since the previous 2009 guideline, which, along with significant social and economic changes impacting on the experience of depression and delivery of treatments, clearly merits a new assessment of evidence. Yet, it is critical that any new guideline takes a properly balanced and nuanced approach to evidence synthesis combined appropriately with service user views, given the potential impact it will have on commissioning in the UK and further afield (several European guidelines as well as Canadian guidelines look towards NICE as the authoritative model). Elements of the first 2004 guideline on depression were employed with huge success as a lobbying device to dramatically change the nature and shape of the psychological therapy workforce and delivery in the form of the Improving Access to Psychological Therapy (IAPT) programme. In spite of many stakeholder concerns at that time about the narrow focus of IAPT on Cognitive Behavioural Therapy (CBT), the combination of NICE's skewed methodological approach and lobbying by professional groups with significant support from influential politicians, led to a significant increase in CBT training and provision, whereas training and delivery of other therapies decreased, significantly reducing patient choice.

This paper sets out key concerns regarding the methodology employed to date in the draft guideline, indicating that the guideline will not be fit for purpose and has the potential to seriously impede patient choice. Specifically, stakeholders and commissioners of mental health services require treatment recommendations that address the clinical needs of the entire spectrum of patients who experience depression. We argue that alongside the high prevalence of mild to moderate cases of depression, services also face the significant clinical challenge of treating cases of chronic, recurrent, refractory depressive symptoms that commonly co-occur with other morbid physical and mental health conditions. If adopted without significant redesign, these issues will have a major impact on care for a significant proportion of the population given that, although not everyone experiencing depression will have a formal diagnosis, 42% of adults report experiencing depression at some time in their life (Mental Health Foundation, n.d.). The guideline will impact individuals, families and communities as well as people in other nations that have in the past adopted NICE guidelines. The largest impact will be felt as a result of not adequately meeting the challenges of chronic, recurrent and complex cases.

In this paper, we address a number of key issues with the draft guideline and illustrate how these issues impact significantly on the way recent RCTs for chronic depression (CD), treatment resistant depression (TRD) and complex depression have been classified in the draft guideline, leading to a bias against psychological therapies generally and psychodynamic psychotherapies in particular. The focus on CD and TRD is chosen partly because of the limited availability of effective interventions for this group who are therefore already disadvantaged by current services and likely to be most affected by any implementation of the guideline. Because of the focus on TRD and CD, in the more technical aspects of critique, we draw mainly on two recent RCTs of psychodynamic psychotherapy for TRD. These are Fonagy et al. (2015), an RCT of 18-month individual long-term psychodynamic psychotherapy (LTPP) for TRD with a two-year follow-up; and Town, Abbass, Stride, and Bernier (2017), an RCT of short-term psychodynamic psychotherapy (STPP) for TRD with an average of 16 sessions and one-year follow-up.

Undermining subjective experience

NICE made a decision not to update the section in the guideline on service user experience purportedly because of insufficient stakeholder responses supporting an update during the scoping phase of development. This is regrettable given that the section copied over from the 2009 guideline (NICE, 2009) was inadequate. Experience of depression is intertwined with the social and economic context in which people live. It relates to levels of community cohesion, economic circumstances, social support and loneliness. There is growing evidence of the impact of austerity on depression and many clients with depression have been significantly affected by reductions in their benefits, loss of work or changes to employment conditions resulting from the economic downturn and political choices (see for example Psychologists Against Austerity, n.d.). Experiences of depression will have been affected by this and there is no scientific basis for the assumption that experience of depression is a static biological phenomenon (see, for example Kendler, 2016). There have also been changes which impact on the extent to which stigma features in client experience. Campaigns such a Time to Change (Henderson et al., 2016) may (or may not) have had an impact on the experience of depression and help seeking. Recent policy changes could also have impacted on experiences of carers; the Care Act coming into law in 2014 and benefit changes mean that carers' experiences are unlikely to be the same as in 2004 or 2009. The guideline approach implies these have remained largely static.

The 2009 Guideline Committee (GC) reviewed some primary qualitative literature but the review was based on one existing review of patient experience of guided self-help for depression (Khan, Bower, & Rogers, 2007) plus two other articles. This focus is skewed and narrow. There is a great deal of primary research on experiences of depression and experiences of treatments going well beyond guided self-help interventions. The review by the GC (transferred verbatim from the 2009 version) is therefore muddled and incomplete. Recent literature since 2009 (not reviewed by the GC) extends client experience data to under-represented groups and has been undertaken in more recent social and economic contexts (e.g. Anderson & Roy, 2013; Brown et al., 2012; Bryant-Bedell & Waite, 2010; Corcoran et al., 2013; Gask, Aseem, Waquas, & Wahid, 2011; Körner et al., 2011; Oliffe, Han, Ogrodniczuk, Phillips, & Roy, 2011; Oliffe, Ogrodniczuk,

Bottorff, Johnson, & Hoyak, 2012; Oliffe et al., 2013; Patterson-Kane & Quirk, 2014; Smith & Rhodes, 2015; van Grieken et al., 2014). Recent literature also includes a qualitative metasynthesis of the experiences of people caring for partners or family members with depression (Priestley & McPherson, 2016) which could have informed the current guideline. There have also been many case studies published (for example Cohen, 2016; Roberts & Sedley, 2016).

Leaving aside the neglect of recent evidence, patient experience data that were used in the 2009 guideline consisted of seven written accounts collected by the GC and a reanalysis of 38 individual accounts extracted from an online database 'Healthtalkonline'. The seven service user accounts were written by respondents who were asked to compose a written narrative considering a set of closed questions. It is unclear how diverse the sample was, nor what formal method of analysis if any was used. The guideline printed the accounts in full and provided a very brief summary of their content:

> Although the 6 questions were aimed at people with any form of depression, all of the personal accounts received were from people who have/have had severe and chronic depression, spanning many years. The themes that are most frequently expressed in the testimonies include trauma or conflict in childhood as a perceived cause of depression; the need for long-term psychotherapy for people with severe and chronic depression; the need to take personal responsibility for and understand the illness to improve outcomes; issues around diversity; paid and unpaid employment as an important part of the recovery process; the negative impact on daily functioning; concerns regarding stigma and discrimination in the workplace; and the relationship between people with depression and professionals. (p. 68)

This analysis lacks depth and rigour but more importantly, these findings were not incorporated into methodological approaches in the guideline or treatment recommendations. The 2009 review also re-analysed 38 accounts from a secondary data source (Healthtalkonline). No demographic details were given for the individuals whose accounts were taken from the database so it is unclear which elements of the population were represented in the data selected. The extent to which the Healthtalkonline data or the seven personal accounts collected included under-represented populations such as BAME, men, older adults, non-heterosexual clients is unclear.

Given the purpose of a NICE review is to review existing evidence, a full systematic review of primary studies in this field employing formal methodology for synthesis such as meta-ethnographic synthesis (Noblit & Hare, 1988), metasummary (Sandelowski & Barroso, 2003) or narrative synthesis (Popay et al., 2006) would have been a more appropriate approach to a guideline review. This would have enhanced understanding of service user experiences, a position held by several bodies including the American Psychiatric Association (2006), the Cochrane Collaboration (Noyes, Popay, Pearson, Hannes, & Booth, 2011) and the Health Foundation (2017). Review of qualitative findings should also be incorporated into treatment recommendations rather than being left as a stand-alone section. As to how this limitation has already disadvantaged psychodynamic psychotherapy, the guideline notes:

> There was a strong feeling within the service user and carer topic group that … psychological treatment offered by the NHS in the form of CBT does not go far enough in addressing the trauma experienced in childhood. The study by Ridge and Ziebland (2006) confirms the opinions of the topic group and the testimony from the personal accounts that people with 'deep and complex problems felt the need for longer term therapy'. Those that have had long-term psychodynamic therapy report that it has been helpful in their understanding of themselves and their depression and that until they have worked through and repaired the damage experienced in childhood, depression will be a major factor in the person's life. The service user and carer topic group do acknowledge, however, that as there has been little research into the efficacy of long-term psychodynamic therapy, it cannot be recommended as a course of treatment in this guideline. (p. 97)

This comment was made around 10 years ago. Since then studies have been carried out on psychodynamic psychotherapies for long-term depression (e.g. Fonagy et al., 2015; Town et al., 2017, both discussed below). None of the recommendations (p. 100) deriving from service user and carer experiences relate to interventions and the guideline makes no policy comment about the key issue raised by service users and carers concerning stigma, which effects their help seeking behaviour even before any treatment choice is considered. Many of the new recommendations throughout the guideline do nod towards patient choice by recommending that if the patient 'does not want' the treatment recommended, an alternative (from a specified list) should be offered. This is, however, a limited interpretation of patient choice and fails to acknowledge inequity of access to a range of therapies as a result of the impact of the previous guideline. Any new guideline should be informed by an impact assessment of the previous guideline and this missing step has led to inequity of access to therapies compounding NICE's limited commitment to patient choice.

Erroneous classification of depression subtypes and bona fide treatments

Depression is an extremely diverse presentation, not least in terms of chronicity, severity and complexity. Treatments are also very diverse and inevitably, RCTs of treatments for depression have a wide range of designs, measures and analytic approaches. The task of a systematic review team is therefore hugely complex, an exercise in comparing apples and pears on a mammoth scale. In order to remain within the restrictions of a diagnostic paradigm with a strict evidence hierarchy, some blunt categorical decisions must be made. However, although the GC acknowledges that there are considerable problems when attempting to classify depression and thus trials into categories, the approach to classification in this draft guideline is concerning. We examine the classifications the GC use for severity, complexity and chronicity and how these impact on their handling of psychodynamic psychotherapy RCTs. We also illustrate how the incorrect categorisation of psychodynamic psychotherapies leads to selective exclusion of bona fide treatments and selective inclusion of non bona fide treatments, all of which leads to unreliable analyses and conclusions.

An idiosyncratic approach to depression severity

The draft guideline used a method of dividing trial populations by dichotomising baseline severity as 'more severe' or 'less severe'. This single reductive proxy estimate of severity depends on the un-evidenced assumption that the equivalence algorithm combining different depression rating scales developed by the GC is reliable and valid. Most of the component measures take into account their own range of severity categories, validated in the literature. The decision to ignore these risks misrepresenting the true severity of a study population and thus forming inaccurate judgements on the effectiveness of treatments. For instance, the study populations in the Fonagy et al. (2015) and Town et al. (2017) RCTs of LTPP and STPP, respectively, are both categorised as 'Less severe' for baseline severity. Fonagy et al. (2015) and Town et al. (2017) used the 17-item Hamilton Depression rating scale (HAMD) and according to the HAMD validated categories, the mean baseline scores for both studies fell in the 'severe' range. This indicates a significant discrepancy between the guideline method and the method established in the literature.

The GC approach to severity also fails to take account of individual change and amount of change. It is more difficult for a treatment to move an individual from a very high score on a measure to the target low score which would count as 'full remission'. It is easier to move someone into full remission if they start on or closer to the low score one has to reach to count as being in remission. It would therefore have been important for the guideline to look at rates of partial remission as well as full remission, particularly where participants begin the intervention with severe depression.

It would be yet more useful to look at individual change. There is significant variation in individual baseline severity scores within and between studies. Examining Standardised Mean Differences alone is an inadequate approach to looking at change. A method for determining Reliable and Clinically Significant Change for each participant individually (Jacobson & Truax, 1991) offers a better assessment of how changes on different measures taking individual baseline severity into account might be interpreted. This method is employed in IAPT reports in which recent figures show an overall 'recovery' rate of 46.3% (Health & Social Care Information Centre [HSCIC], 2016). IAPT reports then examine 'reliable improvement' (which considers baseline and end-point severity, rather than only whether the case met 'clinical caseness' at either point). This finds that 62.2% of IAPT clients improve – a higher figure than when just reporting % reaching the 'recovery' point. Using 'reliable improvement' methods in the trials included in the guideline meta-analyses would offer a fuller picture, which is particularly important when trials have studied the treatment of markedly severe and refractory populations for whom currently there are few well-evidenced treatments available.

Chronicity: mistaken augmentation strategies

The draft guideline separates RCTs of CD and TRD into two discrete categories, whether or not study populations fell into both categories. RCTs that fit both categories were allocated to one category or the other with no explicit criterion for deciding which category takes precedence. The 2009 guideline noted that the overlap of CD and TRD populations is so large as to render questionable their separation as a means of structuring meta-analyses and therefore did not use the TRD category. The 2009 guideline cited evidence for a more loosely defined heterogenous group of long-term, difficult-to-treat depressive conditions, frequently associated with dysthymia and co-morbid common mental disorders, various personality traits and serious psychosocial disability. This position is also followed by the APA in the fifth edition of the Diagnostic and Statistical Manual (DSM, 2013) and the European Psychiatric Association guidelines for persistent depression (EPA; Jobst et al., 2016).

The separation of CD and TRD in NICE's draft guideline gives rise to considerable confusion. The definition of treatment resistance given states that a study should include people 'who have not tolerated previous treatment (for the current episode), and who have been randomised to the further line interventions at the point at which they had no/adequate/limited response' (p. 343). This definition requires studies to prospectively monitor responses to treatments prior to allocating participants to a study of TRD. The definition of CD is based on a retrospective judgement; studies must meet 'criteria for full Major Depressive Disorder (MDD) for 2 years; persistent subthreshold symptoms (dysthymia); double depression (an acute episode of MDD superimposed on dysthymia)'. Many subjects in the trials included in the TRD meta-analysis will also meet the definition of CD. Ruhe, van Rooijen, Spijker, Peeters, and Schene (2012) note: 'because of their chronic clinical course, approximately 40% of CD patients also fulfil criteria for TRD ...... usually defined by the number of non-successful biological treatments'.

The definitions given of TRD in the guideline (pp. 342–343) are exclusively pharmacological requiring operationalisation of dose and duration monitoring. They are not those used in usual clinical settings where case identification is usually descriptive and involves complex evaluations of psychosocial functioning across several domains. They imply that the inadequate response to the agent was immediately recent or current. Trials in this category are classed as 'dose escalation' or 'augmentation strategies', the latter including various sub-types such as augmenting with another antidepressant; augmenting with a psychological intervention, etc. Both the Fonagy et al. (2015) study of LTPP and the Town et al.

(2017) study of STPP were classified as trials of 'augmenting the antidepressant with a psychological intervention versus continuing with the antidepressant only'. Other trials classed as TRD generally established TRD by means of a medical model operationalisation. For example, the Kocsis et al. (2009) criteria read:

> Inadequate response to 12 weeks of antidepressant medication according to a pharmacotherapy algorithm. Inadequate response defined as failing to meet criteria for remission (≥60% reduction in HAMD score, a HAMD total score <8, and no longer meeting DSM-IV criteria for MDD for 2 consecutive visits during weeks 6 through 12). (Table 120)

While the participants in the LTPP study are described by the authors as 'treatment resistant', participants do not meet the criteria for TRD defined by NICE and the intervention was not an 'augmentation strategy'. The criteria were broadly inclusive, stating participants should have had an 'Inadequate response to least two different treatments (mean of 3.7 previously failed treatment attempts)' (Fonagy et al., 2015). This represents a fundamentally different approach to 'resistance'. There was no requirement in the inclusion criteria that the medication received need be recent or current. Although the appendices of the guideline indicate that the study met criteria for CD as well as TRD, it is analysed along with other TRD studies. It is similarly misleading to classify Town et al. (2017) as an augmentation strategy, particularly given that two-thirds in the STPP group reduced or came off medication while just over half the control group increased or started medication. Conceiving of these studies as 'augmentations' of medications is clearly a misrepresentation with the consequence that they are then compared directly against drug trials in methodologically inappropriate ways.

Selective inclusion of non bona fide treatments

The recent RCT by Town et al. (2017) provides evidence for the use of psychodynamic psychotherapy for treatment resistant depression. Based upon the accurate inclusion of only bona fide therapies for treatment resistant depression, the evidence for STPP as a first-line treatment approach is at least comparable to that for Interpersonal Psychotherapy Therapy (IPT) which is recommended based on evidence from one low quality single study of IPT in which IPT did not even outperform 'treatment as usual' (Souza et al., 2016). On first glance, it is therefore unclear what standard has been used to justify the omission of a NICE recommendation for STPP for treatment resistant depression.

On closer examination of the inclusion criteria of studies included under the category of 'STPP versus treatment as usual or antidepressants', we identified a significant mistake. Alongside the Town et al. (2017) trial, data for Brief Supportive Psychotherapy (BSP) from another RCT (Klein et al., 2011; Kocsis et al., 2009) were included as data on STPP. BSP is a recognised treatment approach emphasising common psychotherapy factors but is distinct from other psychotherapies given its lack of structure and specific interventions. The BSP manual for this trial stated that 'psychodynamic interventions were strictly proscribed' (Kocsis et al., 2009). It therefore should not be classified as an STPP in this instance. The inclusion of a non bona fide STPP raises serious problems with the integrity of the analysis. The GC concluded that there was no effect of STPP as an augmentation strategy, clearly taking a lead from the Kocsis et al. (2009) trial rather than Town et al. (2017) – the latter a bona fide STPP treatment indicating a clinically important and statistically significant benefit of individual STPP. If NICE apply the same standard for evaluating treatments for resistant depression across psychological therapies, revision to the draft guidelines is required in order to include STPP as a treatment option.

The narrow gaze of complexity and exclusion of bona fide treatments

The GC also introduced another category of 'depression with co-morbidites', as distinct from CD and TRD (p. 585). Within this category are the sub-categories 'complex depression' and 'psychotic depression'. Again, these are not in line with DSM or EPA and create false divisions between study populations. Comorbidity with personality disorder (PD) is the only criterion for 'complex depression'; an arbitrary cut-off of 51% of participants having PD is provided bearing no resemblance to any recognised classification system nor any professional or service user trends. Many studies otherwise classed as TRD or CD would also fit the 'complex' depression category but have arbitrarily been placed in another category. The EPA guidelines for persistent depression (Jobst et al., 2016) adopt a slightly more nuanced approach to complexity in depression that is closer to the complexity generally encountered in clinical services. Complexity is noted in terms of early versus late onset, type of depression, number of episodes, early trauma, symptom severity, patient preference and comorbid personality disorder, and that the type of treatment offered should be individually tailored accordingly (evidence level 4; Good Practice Point). The GC use of PD as the only criterion ignores these aspects of complexity and in doing so denies the reality of complex early lives and experiences of trauma that many individuals within study populations are likely to have experienced.

On examination of the 70 RCTs reviewed at full text for inclusion in the 'complex depression' meta-analysis, the Fonagy et al. (2015) study of LTPP was not considered for inclusion and five RCTs of STPP were considered but excluded (see below). Eighty-five per cent of the Fonagy et al. (2015) study population had one or more Axis II disorder. Participants had high levels of childhood adversity (89% – unpublished data available on request); and high comorbidity: 47% had musculoskeletal problems, 25% had gastrointestinal problems; 91% had at least one other comorbid Axis 1 disorder; 54% were unemployed; the mean baseline Global Assessment of Functioning (GAF) score was 49.1; 45% had made at least one previous suicide attempt etc. Clinically this is a very complex population, as was the Town et al. (2017) sample, yet these trials are classed as TRD only – rather than chronic and/or complex, highlighting the systematic ignoring of individual subjectivities which in many cases are likely to be highly predicated on childhood adversity and trauma.

Five RCTs of STPP were excluded on the grounds that these studies included (i) 'no extractable outcomes of interest' (Abbass, Sheldon, Gyra, & Kalpin, 2008; Vinnars, Barber, Noren, Gallop, & Weinryb, 2005); (ii) less than 50% of the trial population had comorbid PD (Thyme et al., 2007); and (iii) less than 10 participants per treatment arm (Maina, Forner, & Bogetto, 2005; Svartberg, Stiles, & Seltzer, 2004). However, despite the protocol for the review of interventions for complex depression specifying the inclusion of systematic reviews and disaggregated RCT data for this population, published disaggregated data were overlooked for 79 participants receiving STPP from these 5 RCTs (Abbass, Town, & Driessen, 2011). All participants in this excluded group had confirmed diagnoses of depressive disorder with PD and treatment outcome data on validated depression scales were available. Three RCTs of STPP (Abbass et al., 2008; Thyme et al., 2007; Vinnars et al., 2005) were essentially incorrectly excluded based on rationale i and ii. Furthermore, disaggregated data from two further RCTs of STPP (Maina et al., 2005; Svartberg et al., 2004), which identified a true sample of complex depression, were excluded because of less than 10 participants per treatment arm. In contrast, one of the five RCTs included in this review (Liberman & Eckman, 1981, study of Behaviour Therapy) had failed to administer a formal PD assessment and precise numbers on those with an unconfirmed PD diagnosis were not provided. Hence, only a 'best guess' could speculate how many participants in this small trial ($N = 24$) may have had PD. The GC conclude that the evidence base for complex depression is limited in volume having only included five small RCTs. If bona fide studies of therapies are selectively excluded from data analytic approaches to examine the effects of a specific treatment in this way, estimates of within- and between-group differences can be expected to be unreliable and ensuing quality statements and recommendations questionable (Leichsenring et al., 2017). Likewise, including non bona fide interventions as noted previously in the inclusion of BSP as an STPP has an equally problematic impact on guideline recommendations.

We acknowledge that some of these technical issues around categorising trials by chronicity, severity and complexity may appear akin to dancing on a pin head and that perhaps a redrawing of the boundaries would likely open yet new potholes. Yet this in itself illustrates that the scientific methods employed by NICE ultimately rely on a series of multiple complex decisions made by a relatively small group of appointed experts forced to come to a consensus to drive through the guideline development process. There are limited objective facts guiding these decisions and there are so many decisions to be made at each stage of review that there are multiple opportunities for bias and/or error to occur. Cumulatively, the result of these decisions for the proposed guideline update is the continued omission of an appropriate and specific place for the implementation of psychodynamic therapies within the NHS. The aforementioned evidence points to an important place for psychodynamic psychotherapies in the treatment of complex presentations of depression.

We might argue that the paradigm in operation within NICE requires such an extent of ongoing adjustment creating ever-increasing complexity that it cannot sustain itself, as in Thomas Kuhn's idea of paradigm shifts (Kuhn, 1962). An alternative approach may be required which puts patient choice central instead of peripheral and which considers alternative ways of conceptualising expressions of psychological distress, for example, formulation-based approaches or trauma-informed approaches like the recent Power Threat Meaning Framework (Johnstone & Boyle, 2018) published by the British Psychological Society. Such approaches move towards acknowledging that psychological expressions of distress have meaning, can be signposts to what is wrong in a person's life and can be open to change.

Parity with other long-term conditions?

The draft guideline states that 'the aim of intervention is to restore health through the relief of symptoms and restoration of function, and in the longer term, to prevent relapse' (pp. 40, l.31–1.32). It furthermore highlights the high likelihood of relapse or deterioration in patients with depression described under the heading of 'treatment resistance' (Section 8.1.2). In spite of this, the draft guideline does not take account of long-term follow-up. Indeed, it excluded long-term follow-up data that might demonstrate whether the aims of interventions have indeed been achieved.

The choice to omit long-term data is particularly difficult to comprehend in the sections dealing with TRD and CD and is likely due to most trials not collecting or reporting follow-up data. This is, however, not an adequate justification. Calls for RCTs of interventions for depression to include longer term follow-up years after the end of treatment, given the episodic nature of depression, have been made repeatedly (e.g. Goodyer et al., 2008, 2011, 2017; McPherson et al., 2005). According to criteria adopted by NICE as well as the APA and EPA, chronic forms of depression must last for at least two years. Studies included in the NICE review report mean durations of illness as long as 7.8 years (Keller et al., 2000); 7.6 years (Kocsis et al., 2009); and 24.4 years (Fonagy et al., 2015). Given the actual mean duration of illness observed, there is an even stronger case for looking at data from follow-up periods in more chronic forms of depression. Moreover, Westen, Novotny, and Thompson-Brenner (2004) note that many patients who respond initially to treatments will relapse and/or present to other services subsequently. Hepgul et al. (2016) noted that 38% of IAPT attenders had attended IAPT previously, pointing to a high relapse rate in practice for many front-line therapies. Long-term follow-up data are therefore crucial in the evaluation of the therapeutic effects of treatments for depression whether it is already known to have been long lasting or whether it is a first episode that may become long lasting.

On the contrary, most trials in the review have follow-up points of eight weeks or less. Analyses conducted to evaluate the effectiveness of interventions in the draft guideline have taken the endpoint as the end of treatment. Moreover, the draft guideline has selectively omitted follow-up data in the very few trials of CD and TRD with follow-up and observation periods sufficiently long to offer data about the longer term durability of treatment effects. The Fonagy et al. (2015) study followed participants for two years after the 18-month treatment period giving a total observation period of 182 weeks. The guideline has extracted the end of treatment data from this study (at which point no significant differences between groups were observed) and omitted the important data yielded by the two-year follow-up data, which showed a substantial effect (full remission Numbers Needed to Treat (NNT) = 9.6; partial remission NNT = 3.9).

NICE does not treat any other long-term condition in this way. The diabetes (type 2 adults) guideline, for example, includes examination of outcomes ranging from two years up to 10 and over, reflecting the long-term, chronic nature of this condition. The epilepsy guideline and arthritis guideline examined evidence including one and two-year follow-up data and in some cases longer. In order to treat depression, particularly any persistent form of depression, as a long-term condition on a par with long-term physical conditions, it is important for follow-up data to be taken into account. To meet with principles of parity of esteem, where mental health is valued equally with physical health, all treatments deemed to be effective and recommended for long-term depression ought to have demonstrated an impact at least one year (ideally two or more years) beyond the end of treatment. If the effects of the treatment wear off as soon as (or soon after) the treatment finishes (or the long-term effects are unknown), then the treatment can at best be considered a reasonable sticking plaster. Treatments for physical illnesses that stopped working immediately after the end of treatment (or where there was no known effectiveness beyond the end of treatment) would not typically be recommended in a national guideline. The impact of ignoring these issues is that LTPP has not been recommended partly on the basis of the absence of end of treatment effects; whereas because of its long-term benefits shown in Fonagy et al. (2015), LTPP should be recommended as one of the options for service users with persistent depression to choose from.

Assessing methodological quality of studies: strategically inflexible?

The GC employed the Grading of Recommendations, Assessment, Development and Evaluation (GRADE) approach, a widely used method of assessing RCT quality which allocates points for various criteria such as sample size, blinding, analytic approach, reporting quality, etc. Authors of the GRADE system note:

> GRADE is 'outcome centric' in that a rating is made for each outcome, and quality may differ – indeed, is likely to differ – from one outcome to another within a single study and across a body of evidence. (Dijkers, 2013)

In general, GRADE is designed to be used flexibly:

> We don't necessarily report on all possible parameters of a study – for example, whether an RCT was single or double blinded, or the precise method of randomisation used – rather, following a critical appraisal of each study, we highlight the methodological or other issues that we feel may affect the interpretation of the results or the weight that might be placed on them. (http://clinicalevidence.bmj.com/x/set/static/ebm/learn/665072.html)

Yet we are concerned that the team undertaking this assessment has employed GRADE inflexibly and has assessed all trials in the same way, irrespective of whether each criterion is appropriate for the type of trial or intervention being assessed. Assessing the quality of a psychological treatment trial in the same way as a drug trial is epistemologically unsound. For example, it is widely understood that blinding participants and investigators is not possible to apply to psychological treatment trials because a psychological treatment is not like a pill for which you can create another pill identical in all visible ways but with no active ingredient. In psychological treatment trials, the therapy is unique to each individual and therapist pair and involves a unique combination of words exchanged between the two people. It is impossible to create a placebo version of any psychological treatment which will fool participants and investigators. Nonetheless, all psychological treatment trials have lost points within the GRADE system for failing to meet this 'standard'. This systematically advantages drug treatment trials.

Use of the GRADE system ought to reflect the complex endeavour of comparing medical and psychological treatments. More specifically, the review should employ quality criteria which take into account the use of a range of outcome measures, in particular the assessment of functioning in addition to targeted symptoms. Functioning is not only important to service users but is also both directly and indirectly related to health service use, social care costs and employment (McCrone et al., 2017) and could therefore be examined as a proxy for health economic outcomes where these are not available. As Dijkers (2013) has stressed, the quality for each outcome may differ between outcomes within a single study and across a body of evidence. A re-analysis of the 2004 NICE review examining outcomes of measures of functioning showed a different order of comparative efficacy amongst interventions (McPherson, Evans, & Richardson, 2009). Calls have long been made for RCTs of treatments for depression to include alternative outcome measures (McPherson et al., 2005; Wampold et al., 2017) and would be in line with those who have stressed that the disease burden is primarily due to comorbidities and not merely to the additive effects of having more than one disorder (Wampold et al., 2017). This is important not least because the omission stands in contrast to the emphasis of the draft guideline in the introduction, which clearly states: 'Where possible, the key goal of an intervention should be complete relief of symptoms (remission), which is associated with better functioning … For this reason the GC examined a range of outcomes (where available), including response, remission, change in symptoms and relapse' (pp. 40, 1.32–1.37).

Service users often report that the outcomes that are most important to them are their quality of life, ability to deal with problems, being able to take care of oneself, feeling independent, feeling able to communicate with others, feeling able to get about, ability to attend education, work or social events (e.g. Zimmermann et al., 2013). Although NICE has acknowledged the importance of these non-medical symptoms in previous versions of the guideline, it has consistently failed to adjust its primary focus away from symptoms. The current guideline has ignored available data on non-symptom outcomes to illustrate where evidence for treatment effectiveness in these areas exist. If the GC employed the GRADE system to emphasise the importance of long-term outcomes and non-symptom outcomes, those trials that fail to measure or report non-symptom outcomes or long-term outcomes would be rated as lower quality. Instead, GRADE has been used in such a way that a large quantity of narrowly focused short-term trials is given much greater weight than those few trials where broader long-term outcomes are available.

This specifically impacts the way LTPP has been assessed. Fonagy et al. (2015) found clinically significant group differences at two-year follow-up on non-symptom outcomes including functioning (GAF), a quality of life measure and the well-being subscale of the Clinical Outcome Routine Evaluation (CORE) measure. This trial was given no credit for measuring and reporting these important dimensions of experience. Moreover, as noted earlier in relation to end-of-treatment versus long-term follow-up outcomes, the Fonagy et al. (2015) trial was downgraded for quality because '95% Confidence Interval (CI) crosses both line of no effect and threshold for clinically important benefit (SMD-0.5)'. In other words, because there was no apparent benefit at the end of treatment, the trial was firstly misrepresented as showing no benefits at all and further misrepresented by being downgraded on quality for the same reason in spite of significant differences emerging at the two-year follow-up.

The GC's application of GRADE in this way systematically biases against trials where the intervention has a long-term effect rather than a short-term effect. This is worse than just ignoring long-term treatment effects – it is in fact rendering long-term efficacy undesirable. The reason why treatment effects may emerge after the end of treatment in trials of psychodynamic psychotherapy is that the aim of treatment is long-lasting relational change rather than immediate but temporary symptom reduction. The way GRADE has been applied has systematically prejudiced against this kind of treatment from being recommended.

Conclusions

This paper has outlined only a small number of the issues we consider problematic in the draft guideline document, focusing specifically on the impact on psychodynamic psychotherapies for complex and persistent forms of depression. There are many more serious but generic concerns relating to statistical omissions, inadequate reporting and lack of transparency in methodological decisions. In particular, there are serious and unique risks associated with the network meta-analysis approach taken, over and above that of standard meta-analyses that need addressing (Del Re, Spielmans, Flückiger, & Wampold, 2013; Keefe, 2015). It appears that these have not been adequately resolved in the approach adopted in the draft guideline, leading to serious apprehension in accepting the treatment recommendations. In addition, there are concerns about GC choices made in many recommendations to weigh cost-effectiveness above clinical effectiveness and a reliance on statistical significance of effects (assessed in the GRADE system) which tends to create a paradox whereby small effects detected in well-powered studies are used to justify a recommendation, whereas much larger clinical effects can be detected in small samples. 'Underpowered' studies 'contain valuable information when combined with others like them in a meta-analysis' (Hunter & Schmidt, 2004, p. 12). Therapist effects have also been ignored in the reviews in spite of clear and growing evidence for their impact. For example, Baldwin and Imel (2013) found that therapist effects account for approximately 5-8% of patient outcomes.

In spite of several additional issues touched on only briefly here, the concerns detailed and elaborated upon in this paper focus primarily on issues around lack of proper use of service user experience data; problematic categorisations of depression and treatments in respect of severity, complexity and chronicity; inaccurate inclusion of non bona fide treatments or exclusion of relevant bona fide treatment studies when collating evidence for psychodynamic therapies; issues around the focus on short-term symptom-based outcomes to the neglect of crucial long-term follow-up data; and concerns about the system of assessing methodological quality. This is particularly troubling given that there are so few well-evidenced treatments available for these groups of people and thus the approach in the guideline further disadvantages this under-served group and mitigates against them being able to access interventions which may have the potential to help alleviate some of their suffering. Moreover, it disregards patient choice and the increasing preference for psychological treatments over medication by service users (McHugh, Whitton, Peckham, Welge, & Otto, 2013; van Schaik et al., 2004). The brief eight-week stakeholder consultation process allowed many of these concerns to be aired but we would argue that it is unreliable and unsafe to rely on a one-off short consultation process to correct such serious mistakes and, arguably, the time limits imposed on the consultation and subsequent publication period are too tight for NICE to be able to reconsider their approach. NICE and the 'evidence based medicine' paradigm within which it sits have been shaped by medical science and are now in need of a re-visioning which places patient choice, parity of esteem and equity of access at the centre.

Disclosure statement

No potential conflict of interest was reported by the authors.

References

Abbass, A., Sheldon, A., Gyra, J., & Kalpin, A. (2008). Intensive short-term dynamic psychotherapy of patients with DSM IV personality disorders: A randomized controlled trial. *Journal of Nervous and Mental Disease, 196*(3), 211–216.

Abbass, A., Town, J., & Driessen, E. (2011). The efficacy of short-term psychodynamic psychotherapy for depressive disorders with comorbid personality disorder. *Psychiatry, 74*(1), 58–71.

American Psychiatric Association. (2006). Evidence-based practice in psychology. *American Psychologist, 61*, 271–285.

American Psychiatric Association. (2013). *Diagnostic and statistical manual of mental disorders (DSM–5)*. Arlington, VA: Author.

Anderson, C., & Roy, T. (2013). Patient experiences of taking antidepressants for depression: A secondary qualitative analysis. *Research in Social and Administrative Pharmacy, 9*(6), 884–902.

Baldwin, S. A., & Imel, Z. E. (2013). Therapist effects: Findings and methods. In M. J. Lambert (Ed.), *Bergin and Garfield's handbook of psychotherapy and behavior change* (6th ed., pp. 258–297). New York, NY: Wiley.

Brown, A., Scales, U., Beever, W., Rickards, B., Rowley, K., & O'Dea, K. (2012). Exploring the expression of depression and distress in aboriginal men in central Australia: A qualitative study. *BMC Psychiatry, 1*(12), 97.

Bryant-Bedell, K., & Waite, R. (2010). Understanding major depressive disorder among middle-aged African American men. *Journal of Advanced Nursing, 66*(9), 2050–2060.

Care Act. (2014). Retrieved from http://www.legislation.gov.uk/ukpga/2014/23/contents/enacted

Cohen, R. (2016). Getting into the Acceptance and Commitment Theory with psychoanalytic therapy: The case of 'Daniel'. *Pragmatic Case Studies in Psychotherapy, 12*(1), 1–30.

Corcoran, J., Brown, E., Davis, M., Pineda, M., Kadolph, J., & Bell, H. (2013). Depression in older adults: A meta-synthesis. *Journal of Gerontological Social Work, 56*(6), 509–534.

Del Re, A. C., Spielmans, G. I., Flückiger, C., & Wampold, B. E. (2013). Efficacy of new generation antidepressants: Differences seem illusory. *PLoS ONE, 8*(6), e63509.

Dijkers, M. (2013). Introducing GRADE: A systematic approach to rating evidence in systematic reviews and to guideline development. *KT Update, 1*(5). Retrieved from www.ktdrr.org/products/update/v1n5

Fonagy, P., Rost, F., Carlyle, J., McPherson, S., Thomas, R., Fearon, P., … Taylor, D. (2015). Pragmatic randomized controlled trial of long-term psychoanalytic psychotherapy for treatment-resistant depression: The Tavistock Adult Depression Study (TADS). *World Psychiatry, 14*(3), 312–321.

Gask, L., Aseem, S., Waquas, A., & Wahid, W. (2011). Isolation, feeling 'stuck' and loss of control: Understanding persistence of depression in British Pakistani women. *Journal of Affective Disorders, 128*(1–2), 49–55.

Goodyer, I. M., Dubicka, B., Wilkinson, P., Kelvin, R., Roberts, C., Byford, S., … Harrington, R. (2008). A randomised controlled trial of cognitive behaviour therapy in adolescents with major depression treated by selective serotonin reuptake inhibitors. The ADAPT trial. *Health Technology Assessment, 12*(14), iii–iv, ix–60.

Goodyer, I. M., Reynolds, S., Barrett, B., Byford, S., Dubicka, B., Hill, J., … Fonagy, P. (2017). Cognitive behavioural therapy and short-term psychoanalytical psychotherapy versus a brief psychosocial intervention in adolescents with unipolar major depressive disorder (IMPACT): A multicentre, pragmatic, observer-blind, randomised controlled superiority trial. *Lancet Psychiatry, 4*(2), 109–119.

Goodyer, I. M., Tsancheva, S., Byford, S., Dubicka, B., Hill, J., Kelvin, R., … Fonagy, P. (2011). Improving mood with psychoanalytic and cognitive therapies (IMPACT): A pragmatic effectiveness superiority trial to investigate whether specialised psychological treatment reduces the risk for relapse in adolescents with moderate to severe unipolar depression: Study protocol for a randomised controlled trial. *Trials, 12*(1), 175.

Health and Social Care Information Centre. (2016). *Psychological therapies: Annual report on the use of IAPT services, England, 2015–16.*

Health Foundation. (2017). *Healthy lives for people in the UK.* Retrieved from www.health.org.uk/publication/healthy-lives-people-uk

Henderson, C., Robinson, E., Evans-Lacko, S., Corker, E., Rebollo-Mesa, I., Rose, D., & Thornicroft, G. (2016). Public knowledge, attitudes, social distance and reported contact regarding people with mental illness 2009–2015. *Acta Psychiatrica Scandinavica, 134*(S446), 23–33.

Hepgul, N., King, S., Amarasinghe, M., Breen, G., Grant, N., Grey, N., … Cleare, A. J. (2016). Clinical characteristics of patients assessed within an Improving Access to Psychological Therapies (IAPT) service: Results from a naturalistic cohort study (Predicting Outcome Following Psychological Therapy; PROMPT). *BMC Psychiatry, 16*(1), 52.

Hunter, J., & Schmidt, F. (2004). *Methods of meta-analysis: Correcting error and bias in research findings* (2nd ed.). Newbury Park, CA: Sage.

Jacobson, N. S., & Truax, P. (1991). Clinical significance: A statistical approach to defining meaningful change in psychotherapy research. *Journal of Consulting and Clinical Psychology, 59*, 12–19.

Jobst, A., Brakemeier, E. L., Buchheim, A., Caspar, F., Cuijpers, P., Ebmeier, K. P., … Padberg, F. (2016). European Psychiatric Association Guidance on psychotherapy in chronic depression across Europe. *European Psychiatry, 33*, 18–36.

Johnstone, L., & Boyle, M. with Cromby, J., Dillon, J., Harper, D., Kinderman, P., Longden, E., Pilgrim, D., & Read, J. (2018). *The Power Threat Meaning Framework: Towards the identification of patterns in emotional distress, unusual experiences and troubled or troubling behaviour, as an alternative to functional psychiatric diagnosis*. Leicester: British Psychological Society.

Keefe, R. (2015). Correspondence. Heightened risk of false positives in a network meta-analysis of social anxiety. *British Medical Journal, 2*(4), 292–293.

Keller, M. B., McCullough, J. P., Klein, D. N., Arnow, B., Dunner, D. L., Gelenberg, A. J., … Zajeka, J. (2000). A comparison of nefazodone, the cognitive behavioral-analysis system of psychotherapy, and their combination for the treatment of chronic depression. *New England Journal of Medicine, 342*(20), 1462–1470.

Kendler, K. (2016). The phenomenology of major depression and the representativeness and nature of DSM criteria. *American Journal of Psychiatry, 173*(8), 771–780.

Khan, N., Bower, P., & Rogers, A. (2007). Guided self-help in primary care mental health: Meta-synthesis of qualitative studies of patient experience. *British Journal of Psychiatry, 191*, 206–211.

Klein, D. N., Leon, A. C., Li, C., D'Zurilla, T. J., Black, S. R., Vivian, D., ... Kocsis, J. H. (2011). Social problem solving and depressive symptoms over time: A randomized clinical trial of cognitive-behavioral analysis system of psychotherapy, brief supportive psychotherapy, and pharmacotherapy. *Journal of Consulting and Clinical Psychology, 79*(3), 342–52.

Kocsis, J. H., Gelenberg, A. J., Rothbaum, B. O., Klein, D. N., Trivedi, M. H., Manber, R., ... Thase, M. E. (2009). Cognitive behavioral analysis system of psychotherapy and brief supportive psychotherapy for augmentation of antidepressant nonresponse in chronic depression: The REVAMP trial. *Archives of General Psychiatry, 66*(11), 1178–1188.

Körner, H., Newman, C., Mao, L., Kidd, M. R., Saltman, D., & Kippax, S. (2011). 'The black dog just came and sat on my face and built a kennel': Gay men making sense of 'depression'. *Health, 15*(4), 417–436.

Kuhn, T. (1962). *The structure of scientific revolutions*. Chicago: University of Chicago Press.

Leichsenring, F., Abbass, A., Hilsenroth, M. J., Leweke, F., Luyten, P., Keefe, J. R., ... Steinert, C. (2017). Biases in research: Risk factors for non-replicability in psychotherapy and pharmacotherapy research. *Psychological Medicine, 47*(6), 1000–1011.

Liberman, R., & Eckman, T. (1981). Behavior therapy vs insight-oriented therapy for repeated suicide attempters. *Archives of General Psychiatry, 38*(10), 1126–1130.

Maina, G., Forner, F., & Bogetto, F. (2005). Randomized controlled trial comparing brief dynamic and supportive therapy with waiting list condition in minor depressive disorders. *Psychotherapy and Psychosomatics, 74*, 43–50.

McPherson, S., Cairns, P., Carlyle, J., Shapiro, D., Richardson, P., & Taylor, D. (2005). The effectiveness of psychological treatments for refractory depression: A systematic review. *Acta Psychiatrica Scandinavica, 111*, 331–340.

McPherson, S., Evans, C., & Richardson, P. (2009). The NICE depression guidelines and the recovery model: Is there an evidence base for IAPT? *Journal of Mental Health, 18*(5), 405–414.

McCrone, P., Rost, F., Koeser, L., Koutoufa, I., Stephanou, S., Knapp, M., ... Fonagy, P. (2017). The economic cost of treatment-resistant depression in patients referred to a specialist service. *Journal of Mental Health*, 1–7. doi:10.1080/09638237.2017.1417562

McHugh, R. K., Whitton, S. W., Peckham, A. D., Welge, J. A., & Otto, M. W. (2013). Patient preference for psychological vs pharmacologic treatment of psychiatric disorders: A meta-analytic review. *Journal of Clinical Psychiatry, 74*(6), 595–602.

Mental Health Foundation. (n.d.). *Surviving or thriving: The state of the UK's mental health.*

NICE. (2009). *Depression in adults: Recognition and management.*

NICE. (2017). *Depression in adults: Treatment and management*. Draft.

Noblit, G. W., & Hare, R. D. (1988). *Meta-ethnography: Synthesizing qualitative studies.* Newbury Park, CA: Sage.

Noyes, J., Popay, J., Pearson, A., Hannes, K. & Booth, A. (2011). Qualitative research and cochrane reviews. In J. Higgins & S. Green (Eds.), *Cochrane handbook for systematic reviews of interventions (version 5.1.0)* (chapter 20). The Cochrane Collaboration. Retrieved from www.handbook.cochrane.org

Oliffe, J. L., Han, C. S., Ogrodniczuk, J. S., Phillips, J. C., & Roy, P. (2011). Suicide from the perspectives of older men who experience depression: A gender analysis. *American Journal of Men's Health, 5*(5), 444–454.

Oliffe, J. L., Ogrodniczuk, J. S., Bottorff, J. L., Johnson, J. L., & Hoyak, K. (2012). 'You feel like you can't live anymore': Suicide from the perspectives of Canadian men who experience depression. *Social Science and Medicine, 74*(4), 506–514.

Oliffe, J. L., Rasmussen, B., Bottorff, J. L., Kelly, M. T., Galdas, P. M., Phinney, A., & Ogrodniczuk, J. S. (2013). Masculinities, work, and retirement among older men who experience depression. *Qualitative Health Research, 23*(12), 1626–1637.

Patterson-Kane, L., & Quirk, F. (2014). Within the boundary fence: An investigation into the perceptions of men's experience of depression in rural and remote areas of Australia. *Australian Journal of Primary Health, 20*(2), 162–166.

Popay, J., Roberts, H., Sowden, A., Petticrew, M., Arai, L., Rodgers, M., … Duffy, S. (2006). *Guidance on the conduct of narrative synthesis in systematic reviews.* Retrieved from www.lancaster.ac.uk/shm/research/nssr/research/dissemination/publications.php

Priestley, J., & McPherson, S. (2016). Experiences of adults providing care to a partner or relative with depression: A meta-ethnographic synthesis. *Journal of Affective Disorders, 192*, 41–49.

Psychologists Against Austerity. (n.d.). *The psychological impact of austerity: A briefing paper.* Retrieved from http://www.psychchange.org/uploads/9/7/9/7/97971280/paa-briefing-paper.pdf

Ridge, D., & Ziebland, S. (2006). 'The old me could never have done that': How people give meaning to recovery following depression. *Qualitative Health Research, 16*(8), 1038–1053.

Roberts, S. L., & Sedley, B. (2016). Acceptance and commitment therapy with older adults: Rationale and case-study of 89-year-old with depression and generalized anxiety disorder. *Clinical Case Studies, 15*(1), 53–67.

Ruhe, H. G., van Rooijen, G., Spijker, J., Peeters, F. P., & Schene, A. H. (2012). Staging methods for treatment resistant depression. A systematic review. *Journal of Affective Disorders, 137*, 35–45.

Sandelowski, M., & Barroso, J. (2003). Creating metasummaries of qualitative findings. *Nursing Research, 52*(4), 226–233.

Smith, J. A., & Rhodes, J. E. (2015). Being depleted and being shaken: An interpretative phenomenological analysis of the experiential features of a first episode of depression. *Psychology and Psychotherapy, 88*(2), 197–209.

Souza, L., Salum, G., Mosqueiro, B., Caldieraro, M., Guerra, T., & Fleck, M. P. (2016). Interpersonal psychotherapy as add-on for treatment-resistant depression: A pragmatic randomized controlled trial. *Journal of Affective Disorders, 193*, 373–380.

Svartberg, M., Stiles, T. C., & Seltzer, M. H. (2004). Randomized, controlled trial of the effectiveness of short-term dynamic psychotherapy and cognitive therapy for cluster C personality disorders. *American Journal of Psychiatry, 161*(5), 810–817.

Thyme, K. E., Sundin, E. C., Stahlberg, G., Lindstrom, B., Eklof, H., & Wiberg, B. (2007). The outcome of short-term psychodynamic art therapy compared to short-term psychodynamic verbal therapy for depressed women. *Psychoanalytic Psychotherapy, 21*, 250–264.

Town, J. M., Abbass, A., Stride, C., & Bernier, D. (2017). A randomised controlled trial of intensive short-term dynamic psychotherapy for treatment resistant depression: The Halifax depression study. *Journal of Affective Disorders, 214*, 15–25.

van Grieken, R. A., Beune, E. J., Kirkenier, A. C., Koeter, M. W., van Zwieten, M. C., & Schene, A. H. (2014). Patients' perspectives on how treatment can impede their recovery from depression. *Journal of Affective Disorders, 167*, 153–159.

van Schaik, D. J., Klijn, A. F., van Hout, H. P., van Marwijk, H. W., Beekman, A. T., de Haan, M., & van Dyck, R. (2004). Patients' preferences in the treatment of depressive disorder in primary care. *General Hospital Psychiatry, 26*(3), 184–189.

Vinnars, B., Barber, J., Noren, K., Gallop, R., & Weinryb, R. (2005). Manualized supportive-expressive therapy versus nonmanualized community-delivered psychodynamic therapy for patients with personality disorders: Bridging efficacy and effectiveness. *American Journal of Psychiatry, 162*(10), 1933–1940.

Wampold, B. E., Fluckiger, C., Del Re, A. C., Yulish, N. E., Frost, N. D., Pace, B. T., … Hilsenroth, M. J. (2017). In pursuit of truth: A critical examination of meta-analyses of cognitive behavior therapy. *Psychotherapy Research, 27*(1), 4–32.

Westen, D., Novotny, C. M., & Thompson-Brenner, H. (2004). The empirical status of empirically supported psychotherapies: Assumptions, findings, and reporting in controlled clinical trials. *Psychological Bulletin, 130*, 631–663.

Zimmermann, T. M., Clouth, J., Elosge, M., Heurich, M., Schneider, E., Wilhelm, S., & Wolfrath, A. (2013). Patient preferences for outcomes of depression treatment in Germany: A choice-based conjoint analysis study. *Journal of Affective Disorders, 148*(2–3), 210–219.

OPEN ACCESS

The interpersonal structure of depression

Matthew Ratcliffe

This paper addresses the manner in which alterations of interpersonal experience are (a) central to most of those predicaments labelled as 'depression', and (b) inextricable from other, seemingly distinct depression-symptoms. I sketch an approach inspired by the phenomenological tradition of philosophy, which emphasizes how depression-experiences involve profound changes in one's sense of *possibility*. In so doing, I show how anticipated and actual interactions with other people shape and re-shape experience of the wider world by imbuing it with certain distinctive types of possibility. It follows from this that a shift in how one anticipates, experiences, and relates to other people in general also amounts to a shift in the types of possibility offered by the world. My discussion is concerned primarily with the structure of depression-experiences, rather than with causes or treatment. However, I conclude by tentatively addressing some implications for the latter.

1. Introduction

Changes in the structure of interpersonal experience are central to *most* of those predicaments labelled as 'depression'. Furthermore, various other 'depression symptoms' cannot be adequately conceived of in isolation from the interpersonal. However, one can be forgiven for thinking otherwise. Consider, for instance, the diagnostic criteria for 'major depressive disorder' in DSM-5. It is stated that five (or more) of nine symptoms must be present, including at least one of two core symptoms (depressed mood and loss of interest) and others from a list of seven (weight and or appetite changes; sleep disturbance; activity changes; fatigue; worthlessness and/or guilt; lack of concentration; thoughts of death or suicide). Interpersonal relations are not explicitly mentioned at all (American Psychiatric Association, 2013, pp. 160, 161). Granted, persistent feelings of worthlessness and guilt do at least point towards a wider change in how one relates to others. However, its nature is not addressed and, in any case, the presence of such feelings is not essential to the diagnosis. We are thus left with the impression that any disturbances in the interpersonal realm are *effects* of depression symptoms: social relations are impaired because the person is depressed. This is illustrative of a wider tendency to think of depression, and psychiatric illness more generally, as a disorder of the individual.[1]

In contrast, first-person accounts of depression consistently convey the centrality of interpersonal experience. Consider the following excerpt, from a depression memoir by Tracy Thompson:

> I wanted a connection I couldn't have; I did not understand or value the ones I did have. It was a story I saw time and time again in the ward. 'Only connect!' E. M. Forster had written, but we hadn't, or couldn't, or never had. There was the doctor, lost in his personal torment, or Heather, grasping for superficial symbols of connectedness, or Luisa, looking for it through sex. It seemed to me the basic definition of any mental illness, this persistent, painful inability to simply *be* with someone else: It might be lifelong. Or it might descend like a sudden catastrophe, this blankness between ourselves and the rest of the world. The blankness might not even be obvious to others. But on our side of that severed connection, it was hell, a life lived behind glass. The only difference between mild depression and severe schizophrenia was the amount of sound and air that seeped in. (Thompson, 1995, pp. 199, 200)[2]

That is my focus here: an inability to be *with* other people in a certain way. We might be sceptical about the reliability of certain sources of testimony, such as depression memoirs and we should certainly be wary of cursory remarks about the differences between depression and schizophrenia. Nevertheless, what Thompson writes is, in my opinion, broadly right. Other depression memoirs similarly emphasize this inability to 'connect'. For example, Sally Brampton (2008, p. 1) writes, 'If we connect with even one other human being who truly understands, we take one step out of the illness. Life is about connection. There is nothing else. Depression is the opposite; it is an illness defined by alienation'. Furthermore, the theme of painful disconnection from others is not specific to published memoirs; it is just as prominent in almost every detailed first-person account of depression, regardless of source. In what follows, I will illustrate my various points by quoting from responses to a questionnaire study that I conducted with colleagues in 2011. (Unless otherwise indicated, testimonies quoted here were acquired via this study. Most of the respondents whom I quote from had diagnoses of major depression. In other instances, the experiences described are equally consistent with that diagnosis. For full details of the study, see Ratcliffe, 2015). There remains the concern that over-reliance on one source of testimony has its limitations and presents a number of interpretive challenges. However, the kinds of descriptions offered by respondents are consistent with first-person accounts more generally, as is their emphasis on the interpersonal.

I will not speculate as to the causes of depression, even though many people do attribute their depression to sequences of unpleasant circumstances involving other people, often dating back to childhood. Instead, my emphasis is on the relevant phenomenology: on what the experience of social isolation actually *consists of* and how it relates to other, seemingly distinct aspects of depression. It is easy enough to illustrate that interpersonal experience *is* central to depression, regardless of what diagnostic manuals and the like might suggest. But there remains the temptation to construe it as an isolable symptom amongst others. What I want to show here is exactly *how* the interpersonal is integrated into a wider experience of depression (or, to put it more accurately, how it is integrated into wider experiences of the kind(s) that are often associated with the label 'depression' and, more specifically, 'major depression'). My approach draws on the phenomenological tradition of philosophy, which I think is especially well-placed to clarify the nature of the relevant experiences, given its distinctive emphasis on how we find ourselves situated in a 'world'. With this emphasis, I will suggest, we can come to see exactly *how* the interpersonal fits in.

It is debatable whether and to what extent the kinds of approaches advocated by phenomenological philosophers are compatible with one or another conception of psychoanalysis and with wider therapeutic practice. I will not try to tackle this set of issues here. However, I should at least stress that the account of depression and interpersonal experience laid out in what follows does not require the acceptance of any particular phenomenological method and is potentially compatible with a broadly psychoanalytic perspective. My aim here is to provide a framework for conceptualizing certain commonplace 'symptoms', one that has the potential to inform a wide range of therapeutic approaches. Furthermore, a phenomenological approach that emphasizes interpersonal dynamics, rather than just 'subjective experience', is especially well placed to enter into dialogue with psychoanalysis. In this respect, my phenomenological analysis is consistent with certain recent attempts to integrate phenomenological and psychodynamic perspectives (Stolorow, 2013; Throop, 2012).

2. Possibilities

A common theme in first-person accounts of depression is that other people do not understand one's predicament, cannot understand it, or do not even try to understand it. Accompanying this is the acknowledgement that depression, or some aspect of it, is extremely difficult or even impossible to describe:

> I think the feeling of being paralyzed by the depression is hard to explain, as it's hard to explain it to myself.

> The disconnection I feel is the most difficult to convey. It's very difficult to explain to others who have never felt it, that the world looks distorted and imposing and alien, and that I don't have a place in it. It's like being in a bubble with no sound or colour, and a complete lack of familiarity in everything, even in places I know well, like my home. Even people seem very alien.

Being unable to convey one's predicament to others and feeling that nobody 'gets it' are not simply consequences of being depressed. They are integral to a more general feeling of social alienation that is itself central to many depression-experiences. But why do people find these experiences so difficult to articulate? Granted, it could be that depression impairs the required cognitive abilities.

However, those who have recovered from depression often state that it remains difficult or impossible to describe. Although the difficulty may well be attributable to a range of factors, a prominent and consistent theme is that depression involves the profound, all-enveloping transformation of a 'world' that was previously taken for granted, of something that people seldom reflect upon or even acknowledge in other circumstances:

> You know that you have lost life itself. You've lost a habitable earth. You've lost the invitation to live that the universe extends to us at every moment. You've lost something that people don't even know is. That's why it's so hard to explain. (Quoted by Hornstein, 2009, p. 213)

> Most of all I was terribly alone, lost, in a harsh and far-away place, a horrible terrain reserved for me alone. There was nowhere to go, nothing to see, no panorama. Though this landscape surrounded me, vast and amorphous, I couldn't escape the awful confines of my leaden body and downcast eye. (Shaw, 1997, p. 40)

The phenomenological tradition is a valuable resource for understanding, given this alteration of 'world'. How we find ourselves rooted in a world and how world-experience differs qualitatively from any attitude adopted towards something *within* a world are consistent themes in phenomenology. Whenever I perceive *p*, remember *q*, think about *r*, believe that *s*, or imagine *t*, I already find myself situated in a world, in a realm where it is possible to take up attitudes of these and other types. Because the relevant aspect of experience is so pervasive and deep-rooted, it is something that we seldom explicitly acknowledge. What is thus needed is a perspectival shift, whereby 'world' ceases to operate as a pre-reflective background to our thoughts (including our thoughts about the nature of human experience) and instead becomes an object of inquiry. Here is how Edmund Husserl puts it, in one of his later writings:

> Waking life is always a directedness toward this or that, being directed toward it as an end or as means, as relevant or irrelevant, toward the interesting or the indifferent, toward the private or public, toward what is daily required or intrusively new. All this lies within the world-horizon; but special motives are required when one who is gripped in this world-life reorients himself and somehow comes to make the world itself thematic, to take up a lasting interest in it. (1954/1970, p. 281)

My suggestion is that the 'world' that is altered in depression corresponds roughly to the experiential 'world' that phenomenology seeks to investigate. Hence, we can draw on insights from phenomenology in order to characterize something that is otherwise elusive. To do so, we first require a more specific account of what this 'world' actually consists of. Importantly, it is quite unlike any experience of or thought about something *within* the world. The world is not taken to be the case in the same manner as an object of perception or belief. Its acceptance is instead a precondition for attitudes of 'believing', 'perceiving', and so forth. In order to take something to be the case, not the case, or possibly the case, one must already be situated in a realm where some things are and others are not. So one does not discover this world as an object of experience or thought. Rather, one finds oneself practically, habitually, affectively immersed in it.

The nature of this 'immersion' can be described more specifically. Another consistent theme in the phenomenological tradition is the way experience incorporates *possibility* and, more specifically, *anticipation*. All experience is said to be permeated by possibilities of various kinds. For instance, when I look at a cup, it appears *as* something that I *could* see from another angle, reach out and touch, or drink from. Some experienced possibilities are perceptual in nature: 'I could reach out and touch it'; 'by moving this way, I could see the other side of it'. However, others relate to goal-directed activities and involve various types of *significance* or *mattering*. My computer, desk, chair and pile of notes are experienced as mattering in an integrated way, insofar as they all relate to my current project of writing an academic paper. The long list of emails in my inbox, in contrast, is experienced as an obstruction to other pursuits that I am preoccupied with, even as a potential threat to my well-being. Many experienced possibilities consist, more specifically, in immediate *anticipation*, in a sense of what is coming next and how it matters. Anticipation of this kind is not separate from our experience of the actual. Rather, the actual is imbued with salient possibilities. Take the case of watching a glass fall from a table towards a hard floor. The prospect of its shattering and making a certain noise is there, now, as it falls.

Importantly, our anticipation of unfolding events is not atomistic in structure. Anticipatory experience has what we might call an overarching *style*, a cohesive way in which one's situation as a whole is experienced as unfolding. The sense of being situated in the world is to be identified with this style:

> The natural world is the horizon of all horizons, and the style of all styles, which ensures my experiences have a given, not a willed, unity beneath all of the ruptures of my personal and historical life; the counterpart of the natural world is the given, general, and pre-personal existence in me of my sensory functions, which is where we discovered the definition of the body. (Merleau-Ponty, 1945/2012, p. 345)

As this quotation suggests, it can be added that a style of perceptual and practical unfolding is inseparable from diffuse sets of felt bodily dispositions. It is *through* the feeling body that we experience the significant possibilities offered by our surroundings (Ratcliffe, 2008, 2015, 2017a). To make things clearer, consider more localized feelings of practical confidence. For instance, suppose one is giving a well-prepared lecture to a group of interested students, while feeling unusually refreshed and healthy. One's experience of the situation as a whole is characterized by the confident, unproblematic anticipation and fulfilment of various significant possibilities. Of course, what one anticipates can be quite indeterminate in nature. Even so, experience unfolds in line with what is anticipated; it does not conflict with it. When surprises and disruptions occur, they do so against the backdrop of this broader pattern of confident engagement with one's surroundings; they are localized anomalies. Such experiences also involve a diffuse feeling of ease or confidence, something that is not localized in a particular part of one's body.

The next step is to maintain that our more general sense of being rooted in a world similarly consists in a diffuse sense of practical confidence (something that I take both Husserl and Merleau-Ponty to be saying, albeit in different ways). Experience has an anticipation-fulfilment structure, which operates as an all-enveloping backdrop to more specific situational engagements, experiences and thoughts (Ratcliffe, 2015, 2017a). And the crucial point is that this structure is susceptible to change. Elsewhere, I have referred to its variants as *existential feelings* (Ratcliffe, 2005, 2008, 2015). Emotions and moods might be thought of as intentional states with more or less specific contents, such as feeling happy about *p*, angry about *q*, scared of *r*, or in a bad mood about *s*. That being the case, existential feelings are distinct from both. It is only in the context of a given existential feeling that intentional attitudes of one or another *type* are possible. For instance, one can only experience something as frightening in a world that incorporates the possibility of threat, of anticipating something as significant in that kind of way. Pronounced changes in existential feeling thus involve shifts in the kinds of possibilities offered by the experienced world. The 'world' of depression can be characterized in terms of such shifts. There is a distinction to be drawn between tokens and types of experienced possibility. The following description of how things appear upon hearing that a friend will not show up for dinner is an example of the former:

> What I was seeing then was not a green bottle, with a white label, with a lead capsule, and things like that. What I was really seeing was something like the disappointment about the fact that my friend would not come or about the loneliness of my evening. (Van den Berg, 1972, pp. 34, 35)

Here, a particular situation is experienced in the guise of disappointment, insofar as certain specific interpersonal possibilities present themselves *as* unfulfillable. Nevertheless, one retains a sense that possibilities of that *type* remain and can be actualized in other situations. The loneliness is contingent and temporary; other such evenings are still possible. In contrast, people with depression diagnoses often experience the world as bereft of the relevant types of possibilities. It is not just this evening that appears in the guise of loneliness; the world offers nothing else. To find oneself in a different world is to inhabit a different possibility space. This, more than anything else, is what people struggle to articulate. It should be added that labels such as 'major depression' accommodate a range of different kinds of experiences. These include various different changes in a person's sense of the possible, along with other predicaments that do not involve such profound phenomenological disturbances. In most instances, though, 'major depression' does involve some kind of shift in the *types* of possibility that are integral to the experienced world. Such shifts are also describable in terms of an altered sense of 'self'; a unitary change in 'how one finds *oneself* in a *world*' encompasses both self-experience and world-experience (Ratcliffe, 2015, 2017a).

3. Incarceration

Many first-person accounts of depression state that, while depressed, one firmly believes that recovery is not merely unlikely but impossible, that the world of depression presents itself as inescapable, eternal. This should not be construed in terms of a specific belief with a circumscribed content. It expresses something much more pervasive: a loss of certain kinds of possibility from the world. The relevant experience comes in many subtly different forms. However, for current purposes, it will suffice to characterize it in an abstract, simplified way. Take the general possibility of 'things changing for the better'. Even when a particular situation seems hopeless, we usually retain the sense that something in our lives could change for the better, the sense that this *type* of possibility remains. But now consider a world from which the possibility of things changing for the better is altogether absent: nothing is experienced as offering that possibility and one cannot even imagine a scenario where it might. More usually, a sense that things could change for the better is integral to the experience of one's current situation *as* contingent – a sense that it *could* change in ways that matter. Drained of the prospect of positive change, the world can offer up only more of the same or something worse. Hence, one's situation is experienced as inescapable, something that is often conveyed in terms of being imprisoned, entombed, trapped, encased in some immovable substance, or stuck behind a sheet of impenetrable glass.

The relevant experience is temporal in structure, more so than spatial. One cannot 'get out' because the required types of temporal transition are no longer amongst the world's possibilities. The same experience could be described with a number of different emphases. It is a change in how one experiences time: there is no future, or one's predicament seems somehow timeless. It is also a change in how one experiences one's body: no longer drawn in by worldly possibilities, the body is sluggish, cumbersome and conspicuous. And it is a loss of hope: one can no longer summon attitudes of the type 'hope'. Interestingly, people not only offer descriptions that are consistent with this emphasis on possibility. Some also explicitly refer to possibilities and their absence. Here are some representative examples:

> You can't see far into the future so you can't see aspirations or dreams. Everything I ever wanted to do with my life before seemed impossible now. I also would think that I would never get out, that I'd be depressed forever.

> … when depressed I see life as pointless and sometimes cruel. I cannot see any possibilities for change or improvement.

> The world seems pointless because when I am depressed I can't see the world in a positive way. All I see is a place full of suffering which I often feel I would be better off escaping from … I can't think positively.

> When I'm depressed life never seems worth living … I think that my life will never change and that I will always be depressed. Thinking about the future makes my depression even worse because I can't bear to think of being depressed my whole life. I forget what my life is like when I'm not depressed and feel that my life and future is pointless.

> My entire focus is on the negative. I cannot see a positive future. I often find myself thinking I could be anywhere in the world right now, doing anything and I would still be desperately miserable.

> The world holds no possibilities for me when I'm depressed. Every avenue I consider exploring seems shut off.

While certain types of possibility are gone from experience, others may be amplified. For instance, without significant possibilities for meaningful action, one might instead experience everything in the guise of threat: 'There are lots of threats in the world and they all seem to be about to happen, or be very likely they will happen. Loved ones are in danger'. There are many variants but, in all these cases, what we have is a unitary change in the overall form of experience rather than a cluster of separable 'symptoms'. And, having acknowledged this, we can begin to see how the interpersonal fits in.

4. Connection

My central claim is that the loss of contingency from the world, the sense of one's predicament as inescapable, is *identical to* the feeling of estrangement from other people. So you cannot have one without the other. In brief, the anticipation of certain types of relations with other people imbues the world with a distinctive degree and kind of openness and uncertainty – what we might call a sense of there being *self-transformative possibilities*. Where such possibilities remain, one cannot experience one's current predicament as inescapable or one's current perspective as exhaustive. And, where they are lost, the world cannot but be drained of a certain kind of contingency. Although the relevant loss is not exhaustive of depression-experiences, it is what we find emphasized again and again in first-person accounts.

It is important to distinguish two things: (a) a sense of connection that we sometimes experience *during* interaction with other people; (b) the *anticipation* of interactions involving that sense of connection. First of all, I will suggest that (a) essentially involves a change in one's experience of possibilities, something that can be subtle and mundane or exceptional and profound. Second, (b) includes a sense of the potential for this, and thus a sense of one's current perspective as incomplete, open to possibilities that cannot be fully specified in advance.

Various philosophers have noted -in one or another way- how, when we interact with another person, the two parties inevitably *affect* one another in a certain, distinctively personal manner (something that can be especially salient in the context of psychotherapy). This does not demand conscious attention and is not something one can willfully avoid. We are inevitably permeable to one another's influence. Through an interplay of expression, tone and gesture, we solicit various affective responses, and these responses are inseparable from how the wider world is experienced. The Danish philosopher, Knud Løgstrup, describes this as follows:

> By our very attitude to one another we help to shape one another's world. By our attitude to the other person we help to determine the scope and hue of his or her world; we make it large or small, bright or drab, rich or dull, threatening or secure. We help to shape his or her world not by theories and views but by our very attitude toward him or her. (1956/1997, p. 18)

Interpersonal processes thus alter the possibilities offered by our surroundings – both immediate and the longer term possibilities. At one extreme are experiences resembling what Sartre calls shame, where one loses one's possibilities in the face of another: 'I grasp the Other's look at the very centre of *my* act as the solidification and alienation of my own possibilities' (Sartre, 1943/1989, p. 263). However, there are many other ways in which people *affect* one another, and the point to note is that all interpersonal encounters exert at least some degree and some kind of influence, however subtle and trivial it might be in a given case. The relevant experience is especially pronounced and also has a certain, distinctive character in those cases where there is sustained, patterned interaction between two or more parties, involving feelings of mutual connection. Fuchs and De Jaegher (2009) refer to an experience of 'mutual incorporation', where the two parties form a coupled system; the interaction between them structures both their understanding of each other and also how they experience their shared surroundings. Complementing this, Fuchs (2013) describes a kind of 'bodily resonance' that shapes interpersonal interaction, fostering a sense of connection in ways that shape wider experience and thought.

Such phenomenological claims are complemented by other sources of evidence, including various empirical scientific studies. A substantial body of evidence indicates that actual and anticipated interactions with others, and even the mere presence of others, influence the perceptual and practical salience of one's surroundings in a pre-reflective fashion (e.g. Bayliss, Frischen, Fenske, & Tipper, 2007; Becchio, Bertone, & Castiello, 2008; Sebanz, Bekkering, & Knoblich, 2006; Sebanz & Knoblich, 2009). Others have proposed that certain regulatory processes are not internal to the human organism but interpersonally distributed. Bereavement and other circumstances can thus involve the 'withdrawal of specific sensorimotor regulators', something that may impact dramatically on how a person experiences and interacts with her surroundings (Hofer, 1984, p. 188). Also of relevance is a substantial and fast-growing body of literature on emotion regulation (e.g. Gross, 1999, 2001, 2014). Regardless of how we might think of 'emotion', it at least seems safe to say that emotions are involved in experiences of significance and salience (and, by implication, experiences of possibility). It can be added that, even in adulthood, emotion-regulation is not a wholly internalized process. We interact with the social environment in a range of ways that serve to regulate our emotions (Colombetti & Krueger, 2015; Krueger, 2018). In particular, interactions with other people play a key role (Diamond & Aspinwall, 2003; Gross, 2014). They can nurture or fail to nurture feelings of connection, which are themselves prerequisites for other kinds of emotional change that shape one's relationship with the surrounding environment (Ratcliffe, 2017a).

All of this is consistent with a variety of mundane, everyday experiences. An example I often find myself using in conference presentations is that of two different scenarios that can unfold when you take a visiting speaker out for dinner after a talk. In scenario A, the two of you 'hit it off' straightaway and the conversation glides effortlessly from one topic to the next. As you walk home afterwards, your world seems enriched – it offers all sorts of possibilities, some more determinate than others, that you had not anticipated before the encounter and perhaps could not have anticipated without it. In contrast, in scenario B, the whole evening is characterized by mutual awkwardness – there is no flow of word, gesture, or expression; points are not followed up or developed; and, after a while, everything seems effortful, difficult. The same restaurant now appears small, suffocating, drained of possibility. And, as one heads home, everything seems somehow depleted, diminished.

Interactions with other people can thus shape and re-shape, in various ways, the wider possibilities offered by our surroundings. Importantly, these include self-transformative possibilities of a kind that cannot be anticipated in a determinate way. Turning to (b), it can be added that, in anticipating interaction with others, what we anticipate includes the potential for such relations (which is not to suggest that we ordinarily conceptualize or articulate it as such). What we anticipate from the interpersonal is distinctive in kind; it is essentially indeterminate, to some degree unpredictable. (This is not to make the strong claim that *only* other people can ever offer certain types of possibility. Rather, the proposal is that there is a qualitative difference between the kinds of possibility *ordinarily* offered by other people and those *ordinarily* offered by inanimate entities and non-human organisms.) It is partly for this reason that we frequently seek consolation from trusted others when bad things happen. Interaction with them can involve re-construing the significance of relevant events, in ways that often cannot be accomplished alone and are not merely a matter of obtaining concrete opinions, advice, or practical support. Other people thus imbue the world with a distinctive degree and kind of openness and spontaneity, a sense that *this is not all there is,* that the possible is not exhausted by those concrete alternatives that I am currently able to entertain. This is something that our experience of the world more usually takes for granted, but it is notably absent in many cases of 'depression'. This absence is central to the relevant experiences.

Granted, loss of possibility in depression can extend beyond what is implied by a loss of interpersonal connection. Arguably, one does not have to be capable of anticipating interpersonal connection in order to anticipate enjoying an ice cream. A loss of anticipated pleasure can thus be further-reaching. Nevertheless, many other aspects of depression-experience *are* implied by loss of connection: a loss of possibilities from the world more generally (including all of those anticipated pleasures that *do* implicate interpersonal connection in some way); a sluggishness associated with practical disengagement from the world; a change in the sense of time, involving a loss of openness from the future; loss of a hopeful attitude towards the future. Conversely, *without* this disconnection, the world *could not* incorporate the profound loss of possibility, hope, and an open future that many people with depression diagnoses describe.

5. Disconnection

First-person accounts of 'depression' are in many respects quite varied. This should come as no surprise – the kinds of criteria employed to diagnose depression, along with more specific categories of depression, are cursory and permissive. Hence, they are highly unlikely to identify a single, unitary phenomenon. Nevertheless, a consistent theme in almost all accounts is the intimate connection between loss of possibilities from the world and an absence of interpersonal connection. Although many accounts refer to an impenetrable barrier between self and others, the experience is seldom just that of being cut off, unable to make contact. Along with this, other people often continue to present certain other possibilities, such as threat, disapproval, condemnation, or humiliation. In all cases, though, what is diminished or altogether lacking is a sense of the potential for a certain type of interpersonal connection:

> I feel less connected to people around me – completely alone even in a crowd … They seem more distant and collectively living their lives around me, as if I am not an active participant in my life.

> I assume my family dislikes me and that everyone is looking at me and thinking what a terrible person I am. I begin to feel as if my friends aren't real and secretly they see what I see in myself which is horrible.

> I would sometimes describe it as though I was wearing tinted glasses when I was feeling depressed. My best friends and family could appear to be enemies, I would fear them sometimes, that they would hurt me, that they no longer liked me. Or, I would, when trying to drag myself out of those feelings make them appear vulnerable, that it was in fact me that could hurt them, and that I needed to protect them

> from my thoughts and actions, I would then distance myself, which would make it even harder to feel better.

There is often an emphasis on one's own inadequacy, worthlessness, or failed moral character, coupled with either the threat of other people discovering it or its being on display for all to see. Alongside this, one may dread, fear, or be suspicious of other people in general. In many cases, there is also anger towards others. Sometimes, there is alternation between blaming oneself and blaming others. Indeed, self-denigration often seems to translate effortlessly into criticism of others: I am a burden / they won't tolerate me; I am worthless / they don't value me; I am alone / they have abandoned me; I can't achieve anything / I'm not supported. For example, 'often I feel angry with family and friends but that changes almost immediately to self-loathing that I could think that way about loved ones'. This is reminiscent of Freud's famous discussion in *Mourning and Melancholia* (1917/2005), at least insofar as Freud proposes that self-denigration can amount to a veiled criticism of others (Ratcliffe, 2015)

Interpersonal experience in depression often involves a further tension. It is not simply that interpersonal possibilities are absent from experience. More often, the *felt absence* of these possibilities is itself a salient aspect of the experience. And, in many cases, one *does* continue to anticipate certain forms of interpersonal connection. However, in seeking them out, one is confronted with a world where there is no prospect of actualizing them, comparable to needing a drink in a desert. There is thus a conflict between seeking to engage with and to retreat from the social world: 'I feel lonely if I withdraw but it feels hard to be around people'.

Distinctions should therefore be drawn between various *ways* of being estranged from self-transformative interpersonal possibilities. Someone might no longer seek interpersonal connection, continue to seek it but experience its consistent disappointment, anticipate disappointment but seek out connection regardless, or continue to need connection but find the interpersonal world too terrifying to venture out into. The latter is consistent with something else that is often mentioned, a pervasive loss of more usually habitual, pre-reflective 'trust' in other people: 'I close away from the outside world, I get a feeling of being scared to go out in case I see someone I know. I don't trust the world around me when I am depressed'. When especially pronounced, this may also be described in terms of 'paranoia':

> I am incredibly negative and paranoid – I can't walk around a shop without feeling that everyone is staring at me. I am convinced that everyone hates me. I feel isolated and that no one understands me. I feel as though I have no friends and I am bad at my job. I feel like I'm wasting my doctor's time.

> When I was depressed, I also became much more paranoid. I assumed that if a friend didn't text me back after a few minutes, they hated me. Tiny off-hand comments

> would make me believe even my own mother hated me. I always assumed that the root of this hatred was my awful personality. I thought that the other people in the building I lived in (even those I didn't know) were making fun of me behind my back. It sounds ludicrous now, but that's how I genuinely felt at the time.

Lack of 'trust', in such cases, is not a localized attitude towards however many people. It is an all-enveloping shift in what one anticipates from others, who no longer seem predictable or dependable. This is closely associated with a wider sense of the world as turbulent, unstructured and uncertain. If you cannot depend on other people, then you cannot depend on social norms, items of equipment maintained by others, information they provide, and so forth. Erosion of trust can also extend to the efficacy of one's own actions, to one's bodily functions; to the reliability of one's thoughts and feelings; and to the integrity of one's sense of self. It is here that we start to see a blurring of the boundaries between experiences typical of 'depression' (of one or another kind), 'post-traumatic stress disorder', 'schizophrenia' and other diagnoses. All can be fuelled by much the same form of social alienation, involving the erosion of a primitive, non-localized, habitual form of *trust* or *confidence* (Ratcliffe, 2017a).[3]

6. Implications

What I have said implies that the establishment of interpersonal connection is not incidental to the treatment of depression but unavoidably integral to it, and indeed central (see also Ratcliffe, forthcoming). Establishing and nurturing a sense of connection that someone experiences as absent *implies* the transition from the frozen world of depression to a world that is imbued with meaningful contingency.[4] Hence a pressing issue to address is that of how to distinguish between different forms of estrangement, which may be amenable to different kinds of responses. Consider a case where the prospect of self-transformative interpersonal connection is altogether absent from experience, where the person cannot even imagine such a scenario unfolding. We cannot rule out the possibility that this aspect of experience is veridical, that he really is impervious to certain interpersonal processes. On the other hand, the relevant experience might turn out to be less robust. Regardless of how compelling the sense of certainty may be at a given time, it could be something that waxes and wanes, perhaps depending on situational factors. To put it in terms of (a) the experience of interpersonal connection and (b) the anticipation of this experience, it is possible for (b) to be wholly absent, even though something remains of the capacity for (a). Indeed, it is quite conceivable for someone to experience something as utterly impossible and then to accomplish it with ease, when somehow coaxed into an appropriate course of action. Hence, one issue to explore is that of when and how certain kinds of interpersonal process might facilitate (a) in the absence of (b), in ways that can also assist in re-instilling a sense of (b).

Another relevant consideration is the level of first-person insight that is present. The need to understand what is happening is often a prominent theme in first-person accounts. In the absence of various kinds of significant possibility from the world, a type of curiosity, even an urge to make sense of one's predicament, sometimes remains. People often emphasize the lengths that they have gone to in pursuit of understanding:

> Ever since I realized I probably had depression (long before I was diagnosed), I did all I could to understand it.

> I have read a countless research on the internet and own a couple of books about CBT and anxiety/depression. I talk to my GP, university mentor, and counsellor. I have also spoken to many mental health professionals.

Furthermore, such accounts often display a remarkable level of insight. For instance, they may acknowledge distinctions between feelings of certainty and propositional judgments, distinctions that elude some experts:

> The other thing I really struggle to communicate is how my emotive and rational thoughts interact with one another. I can rationally think 'I shouldn't feel like I am worthless' and still have an emotive thought 'I am worthless'. Describing how those two things co-habit in the mind is deeply difficult, and I have no real words to describe how those things relate to one another. There is not a simple causal relationship between one emotion and one thought, the relationships are far, far more complicated than that, but I struggle to define clearly HOW those emotive/rational interactions go on.

Importantly, such insights into one's condition can also feed into the project of self-regulation:

> I've looked on a lot of websites, I've read books about depression, I've seen various doctors. I feel that my understanding of depression now is quite good. I wanted to familiarise myself with it as much as possible so that I could find a way out. Towards the end of my recovery, while I was at university, I did several projects on depression, because it was something I was interested in, and to find out more about it.

So an especially pressing question is that of whether, when, and how the intellectual acknowledgement that *there are other possibilities* can retain some hold over a person, despite an overwhelming *feeling* to the contrary. Having established that it is a 'trick', perhaps there is some prospect of overriding it:

> We can then see that it is not necessarily REAL what we are experiencing but just another habitual, repetitive experience that has come back to draw us in again. The more time we CHOSE to invest in these experiences the worse we are going to feel. We can learn to recognise that these mental happenings will come back time and time again and that they rarely change their ugly tune at all! Get THIS and you

> are then in a position to say 'hmmm, fuck that...you know today I'm going to give myself a break from that horror movie and clean my bedroom, or wash the car, or anything but that!' There really is a mental training that HAS to go on for people who suffer with depression, and this responsibility is their own and ONLY their own because we are the only ones that can do it and we owe it to our wonderful selves and the lovely people around us to live a good and happy life.

Where there is some potential to erode a feeling of certainty and inescapability via a better understanding of its nature, this need not be a task undertaken by the solitary individual. As applies more generally, other people can assist in nurturing a sense of contingency that is currently lacking. A problem, however, is that the nature of the relevant experience, the loss of possibility and consequent sense of inescapability, is seldom appreciated by others. As noted earlier, first-person accounts often remark that it is both difficult to convey to others and difficult for them to understand:

> The thing about believing that no one really likes me is difficult to convey with any real understanding. I've only recently really started to understand it myself, and I feel like when I do try to explain it to someone they either don't really believe me (or the extent of my feelings) or they think that I'm trying to get them to reassure me that they really do like me (which is not really what I'm going for). Maybe people have trouble understanding it because they actually do like me and find it hard to believe that I don't believe them.

If someone already feels utterly cut off from other people in general, she will be disposed towards experiencing them as indifferent, uncaring, or failing to understand. So it is arguable that the perceived lack of understanding is illusory and itself symptomatic of the depression. There is no doubt some truth to that. Even so, it is plausible to suppose that certain *aspects* of depression-experiences are indeed routinely misunderstood. And what I have referred to in terms of 'world' is the prime example. It is rarely explicitly acknowledged, something we tend to concern ourselves with only when it is shaken. Consequently, shifts in this aspect of experience are prone to being confused with something comparatively superficial:

> Others have often misinterpreted my behaviour as sheer laziness and selfishness. It is extremely hard to explain to somebody who has never experienced depression exactly WHY you are so reluctant to get out of bed.

> The worst was trying to convince people that the problems I had wouldn't just go away if I really were using 'positive thinking'. Basically people considered it to be my fault and that any time I didn't like something or didn't agree with someone else's opinion I was just being negative which wasn't the case. I am a very optimistic person who thinks the best of people by nature.

> I wish there were centres for the depressed, open 24 h a day, somewhere to escape to without the risk of judgement!

Thus, a particular challenge one faces in engaging with someone's experience of 'depression' is that of acknowledging the potential for profound phenomenological differences between the two parties, in a way that might be recognized as such by the other person. The point also applies to clinical empathy more generally (Ratcliffe, 2017b). Various authors have suggested that it involves not so much 'experiencing what someone else experiences' as being open to potentially profound differences between the two parties. In receipt of this acknowledgement, a person may, as Havens (1986, p. 24) puts it, 'light up in recognition of your sudden presence in their lives'; they 'feel found, and not in the sense of found out or criticized.' Margulies (1989, p. 12) similarly emphasizes how empathy requires 'the capacity to go against the grain of needing to know'. Likewise, the task involves *not* imposing the world of the non-depressed upon the world of the depressed, with all the misunderstandings that this would entail.

This kind of recognition can plausibly contribute towards the goal of making recovery a collaborative project. Once some initial sense of connection is achieved, further possibilities for collaborative self-regulation are opened up. For instance, other people can assist in the construction and revision of self-narratives, of a kind that might either sustain or re-shape certain forms of experience. Radden (2009, Chapter 10) distinguishes between 'symptom-alienating' and 'symptom-integrating' conceptions of depression, where the former sees depression as distinct from the self, while the latter takes it to be inseparable. Narratives of both kinds have potential regulatory roles to play, as does their revision. For instance, a self-integrating narrative along the lines that 'I'm depressed because I'm a useless, horrible person who deserves it' plausibly impedes self-regulation.

All of this is, I admit, somewhat speculative. And the points raised in this section require considerable further development, including some account of how they might relate to more specific therapeutic approaches. But what I have at least sought to show is how (a) the structure of many depression-experiences is essentially interpersonal; (b) the interpersonal is inextricable from the overall form of experience; and (c) a sense of certainty and inescapability, central to many depression-experiences, is to be understood in interpersonal, relational terms. To recover from depression is, amongst other things, to recover an openness to certain types of possibility, which are inseparable from the prospect of certain types of interpersonal relations.

Acknowledgements

Thanks to Jeremy Clarke, Jessica Yakeley, and an anonymous referee for helpful feedback on an earlier version of this article.

Disclosure statement

No potential conflict of interest was reported by the author.

Notes

1. The DSM characterization of major depression is problematic in various other respects as well. For instance, it has been argued that it fails to distinguish a range of importantly different predicaments (Ratcliffe, 2015), has undergone an unprincipled widening of scope (Horwitz & Wakefield, 2007), and tends to be mistakenly 'reified' (Kendler, 2016).
2. The reference to E. M. Forster relates to the novel *Howard's End*, Chapter 22.
3. See also Fonagy and Allison (2014) for a complementary emphasis on this form of trust, and for a discussion of its role in social development.
4. Although I consider some of the implications for treatment, I do not address whether and how my account might contribute to the formulation of causal explanations. For complementary developmental approaches that emphasize interpersonal dynamics, see, for example, Fuchs (2013) and Varga and Krueger (2013). However, it should be added that the essentially interpersonal *structure* of depression-experiences does not imply principally interpersonal *causes*; the causal pathways are likely to be many, diverse, and often very complicated.

References

American Psychiatric Association. (2013). *Diagnostic and statistical manual of mental disorders* (5th ed.). Arlington, VA: Author.

Bayliss, A. P., Frischen, A., Fenske, M. J., & Tipper, S. P. (2007). Affective evaluations of objects are influenced by observed gaze direction and emotional expression. *Cognition, 104*, 644–653.

Becchio, C., Bertone, C., & Castiello, U. (2008). How the gaze of others influences object processing. *Trends in Cognitive Sciences, 12*, 254–258.

Brampton, S. (2008). *Shoot the damn dog: A memoir of depression*. London: Bloomsbury.

Colombetti, G., & Krueger, J. (2015). Scaffoldings of the affective mind. *Philosophical Psychology, 28*, 1157–1176.

Diamond, L. M., & Aspinwall, L. G. (2003). Emotion regulation across the life span: An integrative perspective emphasizing self-regulation, positive affect, and dyadic processes. *Motivation & Emotion, 27*, 125–156.

Fonagy, P., & Allison, E. (2014). The role of mentalizing and epistemic trust in the therapeutic relationship. *Psychotherapy, 51*, 372–380.

Freud, S. (1917/2005). Mourning and melancholia. In *On murder, mourning and melancholia* (S. Whiteside, Trans.). London: Penguin.

Fuchs, T. (2013). Depression, intercorporeality and interaffectivity. *Journal of Consciousness Studies, 20*(7–8), 219–238.

Fuchs, T., & De Jaegher, H. (2009). Enactive intersubjectivity: Participatory sense-making and mutual incorporation. *Phenomenology and the Cognitive Sciences, 8*, 465–486.

Gross, J. J. (1999). Emotion regulation: Past, present, future. *Cognition and Emotion, 13*, 551–573.

Gross, J. J. (2001). Emotion regulation in adulthood: Timing is everything. *Current Directions in Psychological Science, 10*, 214–219.

Gross, J. J. (Ed.). (2014). *Handbook of emotion regulation*. New York, NY: The Guilford Press.

Havens, L. (1986). *Making contact: Uses of language in psychotherapy*. Cambridge, MA: Harvard University Press.

Hofer, M. A. (1984). Relationships as regulators: A psychobiologic perspective on bereavement. *Psychosomatic Medicine, 46*, 183–197.

Hornstein, G. A. (2009). *Agnes's Jacket: A psychologist's search for the meanings of madness*. New York, NY: Rodale.
Horwitz, A. V., & Wakefield, J. C. (2007). *The loss of sadness: How psychiatry transformed normal sorrow into depressive disorder*. Oxford: Oxford University Press.
Husserl, E. (1954/1970). The Vienna lecture. In *The crisis of European sciences and transcendental phenomenology* (D. Carr, Trans.). Evanston, IL: Northwestern University Press.
Kendler, K. S. (2016). The phenomenology of major depression and the representativeness and nature of DSM criteria. *American Journal of Psychiatry, 173*, 771–780.
Krueger, J. (2018). Schizophrenia and the Scaffolded self. *Topoi*. Advance online publication. doi:10.1007/s11245-018-9547-3
Løgstrup, K. E. (1956/1997). *The ethical demand*. Notre Dame, IN: University of Notre Dame Press.
Margulies, A. (1989). *The empathic imagination*. New York, NY: W. W. Norton and Company.
Merleau-Ponty, M. (1945/2012). *Phenomenology of perception*. (D. Landes, Trans.). London: Routledge.
Radden, J. (2009). *Moody minds distempered: Essays on melancholy and depression*. Oxford: Oxford University Press.
Ratcliffe, M. (2005). The feeling of being. *Journal of Consciousness Studies, 12*(8–10), 43–60.
Ratcliffe, M. (2008). *Feelings of being*. Oxford: Oxford University Press.
Ratcliffe, M. (2015). *Experiences of depression: A study in phenomenology*. Oxford: Oxford University Press.
Ratcliffe, M. (2017a). *Real hallucinations: Psychiatric illness, intentionality, and the interpersonal world*. Cambridge, MA: MIT Press.
Ratcliffe, M. (2017b). Empathy without simulation. In T. Fuchs, M. Summa, and L. Vanzago (Eds.), *Imagination and social perspectives: Approaches from phenomenology and psychopathology* (pp. 199–220). London: Routledge.
Ratcliffe, M. (forthcoming). Depression, self-regulation, and intersubjectivity. *Discipline Filosofiche*.
Sartre, J. P. (1943/1989). *Being and nothingness*. (H. E. Barnes, Trans.). London: Routledge.
Sebanz, N., Bekkering, H., & Knoblich, G. (2006). Joint action: Bodies and minds moving together. *Trends in Cognitive Sciences, 10*, 70–76.
Sebanz, N., & Knoblich, G. (2009). Prediction in joint action: What, when, and where. *Topics in Cognitive Science, 1*, 353–367.
Shaw, F. (1997). *Out of me: The story of a postnatal breakdown*. London: Penguin.
Stolorow, R. D. (2013). Intersubjective-systems theory: A phenomenological-contextualist psychoanalytic perspective. *Psychoanalytic Dialogues, 23*, 383–389.
Thompson, T. (1995). *The beast: A reckoning with depression*. New York, NY: Putnam.
Throop, J. (2012). On inaccessibility and vulnerability: Some horizons of compatibility between phenomenology and psychoanalysis. *Ethos, 40*, 75–96.
Van den Berg, J. H. (1972). *A different existence: Principles of phenomenological psychopathology*. Pittsburgh, PA: Duquesne University Press.
Varga, S., & Krueger, J. (2013). Background emotions, proximity and distributed emotion regulation. *Review of Philosophy and Psychology, 4*, 271–292.

The active ingredients of dynamic interpersonal therapy (DIT): an exploration of clients' experiences

Venetia Leonidaki, Alessandra Lemma and Imogen Hobbis

The current article focuses on client's perspectives of the mechanisms of change in Dynamic Interpersonal Therapy (DIT), a brief psychodynamic therapy developed for the treatment of depression. Five participants were interviewed and the transcripts were analysed using Interpretative Phenomenological Analysis (IPA). The results point out four subthemes, capturing different active ingredients of DIT: therapy shedding light on previously sealed aspects of self; the relational exchange with the therapist challenging intimate fears; moving towards an interpersonal understanding of their difficulties; and putting the pieces of their lives together into a coherent narrative. Overall participants described an interplay between relational and insight-oriented mechanisms taking place. As part of the former mechanisms, participants reported the development of a secure attachment to their therapist and the provision of a new relational experience, partly via mechanisms corresponding to the concept of transference. Participants reported an increase in insight to have been achieved via an understanding of an interpersonal and emotional pattern as well as via the restoration of a coherent life-story. Processes that theoretically map onto the concept of mentalisation were also reported. The findings are discussed in relation to the DIT and psychodynamic theory about change and to relevant research literature.

Introduction

The upsurge of outcome research measuring the efficacy of psychological therapies in the last few decades (e.g. American Psychological Association (APA), 2013; Smith, Glass, & Miller, 1980) has provided consistent evidence that psychological therapies work well (Lambert, 2013). Outcome studies support the efficacy of psychodynamic psychotherapy (Shedler, 2010); helping this therapy claim a place in national health care provision in the UK, which has traditionally favoured evidence-based psychological treatments. However, outcome studies do not explain why and how therapy is effective, leaving a significant gap in clinical knowledge. This may be addressed by research studying the processes of therapy (Kopta, Lueger, Saunders, & Howard, 1999). The current article presents a small-scale research study focusing on the mechanics of a particular form of psychodynamic psychotherapy.

Process research may investigate therapeutic action from different perspectives. In the study of psychodynamic treatment, the therapists' contributions have traditionally been favoured over the clients' ones (Schwaber, 1996). This may have happened because psychodynamic treatment has focused on unconscious mechanisms of change, which are not necessarily easily identifiable by clients, and because psychoanalytic theory has historically been constructed via case studies which therapists used to draw conclusions upon. The present study engaged with clients' views of their therapy, which could serve as a valuable source of information for a number of reasons. Firstly, clients' views about what worked in therapy may be different from their therapists' respective views (Todd, Deane, & Bragdon, 2003). Secondly, clients' accounts can reveal complex functions of therapy, not previously predicted by theory (e.g. Hamill, Ried, & Reynolds, 2008). Thirdly, the individual's characteristics may determine client's responsiveness to treatment (Fonagy, 2010), in which case clients' reflections may increase our knowledge of how adequately a treatment fits an individual.

Further, in psychoanalysis there are different schools of thoughts and treatment models. In a literature review, Lilliengren and Werbart (2005) conclude that there has not been a universally accepted model of therapeutic action in psychoanalytic/psychodynamic therapy. Thus, the active ingredients of psychodynamic treatment may also vary depending on the exact theoretical model adopted, and studying clients' views could help us increase our knowledge of such different mechanisms. The current study investigates clients' experiences of a brief psychodynamic psychotherapy, called dynamic interpersonal therapy (DIT), specifically designed for clients presenting with depression in primary care, as explained in more detail below.

DIT is a manualised, brief (16 sessions) psychodynamic intervention for mild-to-moderate depression (Lemma, Target, & Fonagy, 2010) which was introduced to the Improving Access to Psychological Therapies (IAPT) programme in England. IAPT aimed to increase access to high-quality, evidence-based, psychological interventions in England's National Health Service (NHS), an approach which favoured cognitive behavioural therapy (CBT), as the model with the largest evidence base (Roth & Fonagy, 2005). DIT was introduced to IAPT because there was also a recognition that a one-size approach does not fit all (Department of Health, 2010), while its development relied on a distillation of the active ingredients of other evidence-based, manualised, psychoanalytic/psychodynamic interventions (Lemma, Roth, & Pilling, 2008).

The main theoretical schools underpinning DIT are that of attachment (Bowlby, 1969/1982), mentalisation (capacity for reflective functioning) (Fonagy, Gergely, Jurist, & Target, 2002), object relations (Glickauf-Hughes & Wells, 1997) and

Sullivan's (1953) interpersonal theory. In DIT, the therapist adopts a fairly active stance and in collaboration with the client formulates an interpersonal-affect focus (IPAF), which captures non-conscious mental representations of self and other, and a non-conscious relational pattern, which becomes the focus of therapy. The emphasis of DIT is on identifying a pattern that is linked to the client's presenting problems and on enhancing client's capacity for mentalisation and encouraging change (Lemma et al., 2010).

This is the second paper derived from a small qualitative study on clients' experiences of DIT. The first paper (Leonidaki, Lemma, & Hobbis, 2016) focused on how clients experienced distinct elements of DIT, such as its style and time limitations, and the changes that they apparently achieved as a result of DIT. The current article engages with the perceived active ingredients of DIT that seemed to have facilitated the reported changes. Although previous studies exploring the therapeutic action in psychodynamic therapy exist in the literature (e.g. Lilliengren & Werbart, 2005; Midgley, Target, & Smith, 2006; Yakeley & Wood, 2011), the emerging active ingredients of DIT may well be different. This may be because of the therapeutic package in which DIT is being delivered, its underpinning theoretical mechanisms or the client group that it was designed for. It could be also because of its explicit interpersonal focus and the employment of mentalisation techniques to help clients with depression and anxiety. Regardless, a greater understanding of the underlying change mechanics of DIT could aid its development and delivery and could contribute to the relevant literature about the aspects of psychodynamic treatment that clients experience as promoting change.

Method

The three authors are all clinical psychologists, with the first author having been a trainee at the time of this study. While the first author had an interest in psychodynamic therapy as well as other treatment models, the second author is a DIT trainer and the third author mainly practises using CBT. Thus, each author has brought a different perspective to this study, which had to be 'bracketed' temporarily to allow engagement with participants' stories. The current study employed the Qualitative Helpful Factors Design (QHFD), a methodological paradigm where new knowledge is obtained by clients directly discussing views of the psychological therapy received. In particular, clients are asked what they found helpful or hindering in therapy and rich qualitative data about change processes is typically obtained via unstructured or semi-structured interviews and/or questionnaires, analysed via systematic qualitative methods, such as grounded theory (Elliott, 2010). The qualitative method employed in the current study was that of Interpretative Phenomenological Analysis (IPA), which focuses on an insider's perspective of a particular significant experience, as taking place in a specific context. IPA, drawing upon phenomenology, hermeneutics and idiography, is particularly suitable for exploring experiences initiating reflection, such as that of therapy. Indeed, IPA engages with how the participants make sense of their own experiences as well as with the researcher's interpretation of the latent meaning of participants' narratives (Larkin, Watts, & Clifton, 2006).

The data collection relied on semi-structured interviews conducted by the first author in service premises, which were audio-recorded and transcribed. The interview schedule covered the following themes: clients' experiences of their therapist and of the course of DIT, the possible impact of therapy on their initial perceptions of their problems and the impact of DIT on participants' functioning and relationships. Throughout the interviews, the interviewer actively encouraged participants' narratives illustrating what they found helpful in DIT. As part of the IPA analytic process, reading and re-reading the transcripts and making reflective notes allowed immersion with the data. Emergent themes were compared across the group, and they were then organised in superordinate themes. Validity check included an audit trail, the third author acting as an additional auditor and peers' feedback.

Participants' recruitment took place in an NHS psychological therapy service which operated using the IAPT model, as described by the Department of Health (2008). The service was in a highly diverse area of London. In accordance with IPA guidelines which aim for a small homogenous sample (Larkin et al., 2006), all participants had completed DIT between 3 weeks and 10 months prior to their interviews and had entered treatment because they had mainly suffered from mild-to-moderate depression. Individuals who had a diagnosis of psychosis or personality disorder, were actively suicidal or needed an interpreter present in the interview process were excluded from the study. Participants were contacted via a letter. Out of the twenty-three potential participants invited in this study, five took part. Although the small sample size may well limit the transferability of the findings, it allowed for a more in-depth interpretative analysis which is in line with IPA principles.

All five participants also presented with co-morbid anxiety. Out of the five participants, three (Alan, Eric and Lisa) had recovered from their depressive symptoms by the end of therapy and two of them (Eric and Lisa) had also recovered from anxiety. Interestingly, participants having achieved recovery or not did not appear to coincide with whether they talked positively about their experience of therapy. A more detailed discussion about how recovery was estimated, and the agreement between improvements in scores and qualitative accounts can be found in the first paper derived from this study (Leonidaki, Lemma, & Hobbis, 2016).

Results

The findings were found to represent four interconnected subthemes which concern the therapeutic processes that have apparently acted as mechanisms of change from the participants' point of view. The first subtheme discusses previously sealed aspects of self that DIT helped participants become more fully aware of. The next subtheme captures how the relational experience with their DIT therapist has apparently helped them overcome previous fears. The third subtheme describes how participants developed a more interpersonal understanding of their difficulties in the course of therapy. The final subtheme deals with how DIT has 'put pieces together', constructing a coherent life narrative.

Shedding light on previously sealed aspects of self

This theme is about processes that helped participants learn about sealed aspects of themselves, including how they relate to others and previously hidden emotions. In all the extracts, participants attribute a central role to their therapist for facilitating such insight.

Alan uses a metaphor to explain this process in therapy:

> It was not that I did not realise what I was saying, but you don't put it in a context- {…}, but she [the therapist] was able to sort of take this situation and sort, sort of give it back to me and say look this is how you are, it's(sighs) like, I suppose it's like a painter who um … who paints your portrait … you look yourself in the mirror and you think you know yourself but when they paint you, you may not like the way that they painted your portrait, but you can see that there is an inner truth to it, which then you can grab hold of

Lisa talked about how discussing in detail ordinary interactions with her therapist enhanced her understanding of her feelings:

> It {DIT} made me more in touch with myself {…} like, I was on the Tube one time and someone was sitting next to me bugging me, and whereas before I wouldn't even think of how something so small could have had an impact on me, then I would tell [therapist's name anonymised] about it and she was like 'well let's talk about that a bit more', so just a little thing, I was more aware of things and just kind of more, like I said, getting in touch with how I feel cause it's something that I've never really, um, done before

Further, Angela, who reported that resentment was 'shutting' her 'down', talked about how she became more in contact with a fuller range of feelings in the course of therapy:

> They [the feelings] have been underlying there and I was denying them I don't know, I somehow was able to, he [the therapist], yeah, he made me see things much clearly, {…} he made me feel hmm [pause] comfortable, he made me feel that I was important, he made me feel hmm, confident, hmmm, and he also [pause], you know he also mentioned that it was not wrong to have all those feelings{…}, you know, anger, resentment, neglect, love, all those things, {…} and then he made me work where they were coming from, what was the cause and, and how I was reacting at that particular time was due to them

Matthew who reported that a 'light switched on {…} in a different room' in his head, a room where he 'never used to be in', described that there was something about the way that his therapist interacted with him that facilitated this:

> There are certain questions that somebody will ask you that will kind of prompt you to give them an answer that you would not usually give them, you 'd have to stop and think about what you are saying sort of thing and aahh … hang on a minute, maybe this kind of thing prompt you … there, there is something in you that needs letting out, but you don't know how to get it out, and then kind of help you along the way, coach you how to get it out subconsciously sort of thing, it's very strange … but it worked, so what can I say?

Eric explains how a dream interpretation resulted in discovering feelings about vulnerable aspects of himself, connected to the perception of his father:

> I was dreaming about [pause] my dad and me … then he made the point that, you know, feeling small is maybe because I see my dad weak like, trying, yes, trying to be, when I said I always try to be strong, I described my dad as a stronger person than me and other things, blah, blah, so he said maybe I look for that image of my dad{…}so he, he found that relationship, feeling small, trying to act like my dad.

The unique relational exchange challenging intimate fears

This theme captures how the client–therapist interaction served as a mechanism of change by offering participants a different relational experience, which contradicted intimate fears or negative expectations regarding themselves and others.

For Matthew and Lisa, the overall process of talking and opening up itself appears to have been a new and important experience. Before therapy, Matthew did not know 'how to get out' what 'needs letting out' but he explained how DIT facilitated him to 'kick this habit' of not talking:

> I don't really say much, but hmm, it was like, he had little questions, and I'd talk, talk, talk, talk

Extracts from Lisa's interview convey the sense that her pre-existing concern about opening up was related to her fear of being judged, which was disconfirmed in her interaction with her therapist:

> Cause I was able to ask [therapist's name anonymised] for help, so you know that, cause before I was, I just didn't feel like I could get it out, but um in the interaction that I had with [therapist's name anonymised] I felt comfortable enough with her to be able to say 'okay' if I can start with you, then hopefully I can take it outside and start with other people and just build on that as well, so that was that, just being able to say 'okay well I've said this' [pause] she didn't really react to it and then she was, 'why did you think I was gonna react?' you know getting me in touch with my feelings

Alan, who elsewhere in the interview talked about having found it difficult to open up emotionally, explicitly discussed the value of the therapeutic relationship disconfirming his initial expectations that this would be a business-like relationship lacking authenticity:

> I could not really understand whether we were engaged in a sort of role play or whether she was being really truthful {…} had a sort of feeling that went to see a therapist was very much like went to see a doctor or you go and see a [sighs] lawyer; you explain your problems to them and they listen but when you are … left, they sort of forget about you {…} and what I experienced from [name of therapist anonymised] was [pause] that I had an impact on her life just as much as she had an impact on … me

Alan discovered his impact on his therapist after finding out that his therapist was 'hurt' following a temporary rapture in the therapeutic relationship.

Having her own space and her therapist's full attention were also new experiences for Angela:

> Because it was all about me, it was *me, me and me* {…} after a very long time I was able to think about myself, how *I* feel, how things affect *me*[1]

Angela emphasising the words 'I' and 'me' in her speech highlight how her having been treated as important by her therapist made a difference. Perhaps the nature of this interaction contradicted her belief that her needs were not important, conveyed elsewhere in her interview.

For Lisa, discussing her feelings towards her sessions with her therapist challenged her beliefs that she had to relate to others in a way that would fit into 'a perfect little box'.

> Everything for me had to be perfect, if not, it didn't work out so it was quite good just to be able to {…} be reminded that everything doesn't fit into that little box, things that are not gonna go according to plan, like with the sessions, I felt that I wanted more and um me and [therapist's name anonymised] talked about it and she was like 'well, why can't you ask for more?' and I was like 'oh I didn't know I could' because everything fit into that perfect box. So it was good just to be able to have that …

Eric is absent from the current theme, as he appeared to carry highly ambivalent feelings towards the relationship with his therapist, which were partly linked to the time limitations of therapy making him feel that this was 'instant help' and not a genuine one.

Moving towards an interpersonal understanding of difficulties

This theme deals with an apparent shift in participants' understanding of their difficulties over the course of DIT.

When participants discussed their initial reasons for seeking help, they offered descriptive accounts of their distress, which appeared to represent their understanding of their symptoms prior to DIT.

What their narratives shared in common was a description of participants' difficulties in symptomatic terms, while the feelings are experienced as incomprehensible or as the result of stressful life events, such as work-related stress or death of a family member. However, elsewhere in their interviews participants explained how the sessions helped them realise how their symptoms were also the result of interpersonal and emotional configurations, which were now perceived as unhelpful.

More specifically, Alan and Eric, described how in the course of therapy they became aware of how their problems had also resulted from them having taken distance from others to conceal their vulnerabilities:

> Dr [name of the therapist anonymised] would say 'Yaa, that's it, that's what I was talking …' [that] I always take some invisible guard. I try to be always ready a hundred per cent, strong like that, but it was not working, I am exhausting myself all the time. (Eric)

> Looking back on it [pause] the stress was basically caused by my inability to tell people how I felt {…}What therapy helped me to realise was that {…} I was so wanting to please, I was so wanting to be seen as being at the top, top, top of the class um… and in fact the more pressure that I put on myself the worse I felt. (Alan)

Similarly, Matthew concluded that his low mood was the result of building up 'things going on' in his head, which he now reviewed as unhelpful:

> It just kind of built up and built up and built up and built up and it was bringing me to a very low mood

> If anything bothers me, maybe I should, I should not just keep it bottled in

Both Lisa and Angela described how prioritising others' needs over their own and trying to please others all the time was where their difficulties had stemmed from in the first place:

> I think it kind of came back to (cough) the way I was interacting with people, um, because I was putting so much emphasis on them and not looking after myself, it kind of, it was draining basically, and then I felt tired and I felt things were missing because I was, I wasn't looking after myself, I was looking after other people and that's something that I definitely took out from the sessions that I constantly, because I was always trying to please other people {…} and constantly putting in so much energy it took it out, it took out energy out of me basically. (Lisa)

Angela felt it was her 'duty' to attend to others' needs, which often resulted in feelings of guilt. Therapy seemed to have helped her to make this link and disentangle emotions previously covered by guilt.

'Then you put the pieces back into place' (Angela)

This theme deals with the process of drawing connections between different parts of life, as well as the emotional impact of this process as described by three participants. They all mention how in the course of DIT there were references to their past, which then helped them reflect on their current emotions and interpersonal patterns.

For Angela, whose main struggle seems to have been with her powerful sense of guilt, seeking the origins of her emotions seems to have helped her question ideas she had about how she should feel and validate her feelings.

> Then we worked out the way backwards as to why I was feeling the way I was feeling, you know {…} the guilt and the frustration and the anger, the guilt comes from the time I was young, you should do things, you are there to do things for everyone and when you don't do it, that is when the guilt comes from and the anger {…} and how it was affecting me, {…}and why I felt the way I did

Alan explained that looking at his past promoted an understanding of the function of his avoidance of relationships and its origin:

> … therefore the way I dealt with relationships was not to have them. My mother and father had died, that was pretty bad, I had friends who died, I had friends who moved away, I had relationships with women, with girls that ended … um, and I started to build a wall, wall around myself because I was so tired of being hurt, and my way of dealing with that was basically not to have relationships at all

In the first theme, Eric had implied a connection between his past relationship with his father and his current way of relating with others. Here he further expands on the significance of drawing connections in the sessions:

> Dr [therapist's name anonymised], he tries to point things that maybe I knew I had in my past {…} We tried to think this problem maybe is because of this, so I had some connection. (Eric)

Although drawing connections between past and present seems to have served different functions for each participant, the promotion of an increased sense of coherence and connectedness is shared across the three interviews. There is also an underlying sense that telling one's story, seemingly serving as reminiscence, is important in itself.

> It was really what therapy to me should be about, which is basically that you gradually talk to somebody, you tell them about your life experience, you relate things from your childhood, from your adolescence, from your adulthood and they piece together the type of person that you are. (Alan)

> Because it's all in the past, it's all jumbled up you know, we are, we were able to unravel that and were able to direct the anger to a different section, we were able to direct the love to a different section, resentment to a different section you know, it's

> like [pause] [sighs] aaah, you know when you get a jigsaw puzzle that the pieces are mixed up, then you put the pieces back into place, that's the way I see it. (Angela)

Discussion

The overall aim of this paper was to present clients' perspectives of the mechanisms of change in DIT, a brief psychodynamic therapy that has been introduced in the NHS for the treatment of depression. Five participants were interviewed and the transcripts were analysed using IPA. Despite the small sample size, the richness and depth of narratives provided an insightful glimpse into the active ingredients of DIT, as experienced by the participants. The results point out four distinct subthemes, each of them capturing different processes of DIT that facilitated change: therapy shedding light on previously sealed aspects of self, the unique relational exchange with the therapist challenging intimate fears, moving towards an interpersonal understanding of the difficulties that brought them to therapy, and putting the pieces of their lives together into a coherent narrative. In this section, the above processes are discussed in relation to existing theories about mechanisms of change in DIT and in psychodynamic psychotherapy in general as well as compared with the relevant research literature.

In his review of psychodynamic theories, Kernberg (2007) makes a distinction between mechanisms that rely on the therapeutic relationship and those oriented towards facilitating insight. Stern et al. (1998) also compare interactional/intersubjective mechanisms with interpretative ones in psychodynamic psychotherapy. In the current study participants have referred to mechanisms that fall into both categories. This discussion will start with those that fall into the arena of relationships before moving to those aiming to increase insight.

The first two themes, presented in the Results section, appear to emphasise relational processes in therapy. Firstly, across these two themes several participants describe explicitly (Angela, Lisa) or implicitly (Matthew, Alan) how feelings of safety and trust in the therapeutic relationship acted as a precondition for them to open up and consequently explore areas of mind which otherwise would have perhaps been too frightening to approach. Interestingly, Eric, who has been the only participant who painted a negative picture of the effectiveness of DIT elsewhere in his interview, (see Leonidaki, Lemma, & Hobbis, 2016) did not describe having developed a trusting bond with his therapist.

Furthermore, for Matthew and Lisa this process of learning to trust and open up in the therapeutic relationship was described to be transformative in itself, as both participants said that they were not used to talk about their feelings prior to DIT. However, this was not the case for every participant. In particular, for Angela, whose needs appear to have previously been neglected, it was her therapist's attention and having a space dedicated to herself which appeared to have acted as turning points. Alan and Lisa, on the other hand, talked about how their interactions with their therapists helped them loosen their defences and as a result have a more authentic experience of being with the other. For Alan, this involved a sense that his therapists cared and for Lisa a sense that her wishes did not have to 'fit into a perfect little box'.

This suggests that the therapeutic relationship in DIT acted as a vehicle of change in two major ways. The first concerns how the safety in the relationship creates the necessary conditions for the therapeutic work to take place. This first function of the therapeutic relationship is well-supported by research evidence (Burns & Nolen-Hoeksema, 1992; Martin, Garske, & Davis, 2000) and is well-recognised across theoretical models (Grencavage & Norcross, 1990; Lambert, 1992), including CBT (Beck, Rush, Shaw, & Emery, 1987). Lilliengren (2014) makes a helpful distinction between the concepts of therapeutic alliance (Horvath, 2006) and attachment (Bowlby, 1973, 1988) and how these concepts apply differently to the therapeutic relationship. She explains that the concept of therapeutic alliance refers to the conscious and collaborative aspects of the relationship concerning shared goals and tasks, while that of attachment regards the emotional bond between client and therapist which may also operate at a deeper level. The current participants' descriptions of feelings of safety and trust in the therapeutic relationship appear to map onto the concept of attachment, indicating that building this bond with the therapist is the first step allowing them to make use of other aspects of therapy more effectively.

The second way in which the participants described the therapeutic relationship having led to change was via the provision of a new relational experience, as more clearly captured in the second subtheme. Interestingly the specific elements of the therapeutic relationship that brought up such change varied among participants and in order for one to appreciate fully how they operated, they have to be placed in the context of individual participants' lives. This fits with the conclusion made by Beutler et al. (2003) that the active ingredients of the therapeutic relationship depend on idiosyncratic factors related to a particular client. This function of the therapeutic relationship as a new relational experience also appears to map onto the concept of corrective emotional experience, defined by Alexander and French (1946) as experiential re-exposure to early difficult feelings and fears under more favourable circumstances, which in turn facilitates change. It could also be understood in the context of attachment theory, which suggests that the attachment to the therapist shapes clients' existing internal working models about relationships (Bowlby, 1988). This type of relational work that was described by the participants appears to fall into the rubric of working in the transference, which in DIT is always in relation to the IPAF. However one needs to understand the concept of transference here as more broadly referring to a greater range of aspects of the interpersonal process taking place between client and therapist, rather than the traditional definition of transference exclusively capturing unconscious feelings and phantasies originating from childhood which are being transferred to the therapist (Westen, 1988).

In addition to the relational mechanisms mentioned above, participants reported insight-oriented mechanisms in DIT which helped them to achieve change. References to these mechanisms are mainly found in the last two subthemes, with the first one dealing with participants' understanding of their problems in interpersonal terms, and the second one with an understanding of how their difficulties fit in the context of their lives.

In the third subtheme, participants' symptomatic narratives about their problems at the time of referral appeared consistent with the conceptualisations of mental illness provided by the stress-vulnerability model of depression (Ingram & Luxton, 2005) and diagnostic systems currently in use in mainstream psychiatry (American Psychiatric Association [APA], 2000; World Health Organization [WHO], 1992). In contrast, DIT considers it vital to understand one's difficulties in the context of the client's personality and the formulation of the IPAF early in therapy materialises this idea. Indeed, DIT appears to have helped participants appreciate how their symptoms had also been the result of relational and affective configurations, such as avoiding coming close to others (Alan, Eric) or prioritising others' needs over one's own (Angela, Lisa). Theoretically, the above configurations seem to map onto the psychoanalytic idea of defences (Bowins, 2004).

Reviewing the past, connecting it to the present, and identifying the origins of their current difficulties were all processes that were reported to have increased emotional and relational awareness for three participants in the final subtheme. These processes echo the idea that clients' narratives restoring the coherence of an ill-defined life story may promote change (Holmes, 2002). In this sense, retelling one's story and inserting non-conscious material in it is seen as an attempt to fill the breaks in the attempted story, which may have been caused by the function of defence mechanisms (Phillips, 1999). Additionally, retelling a story can help to broaden a previously narrow narrative (Holmes, 2002).

An additional process of change is implied in the second subtheme, where participants' descriptions capture a collaborative process of reflection taking place between them as clients and their therapists, which then enables them to 'put into context' how they relate to others (Alan) or 'let out' (Matthew) and 'get in touch' (Lisa) with previously hidden feelings. The above echoes the concept of mentalisation, which could be seen as a mechanism of change which combines relational and insight-oriented elements (Lilliengren, 2014). In therapy, mentalisation refers to the process through which the therapist helps the client reflect on their own and other's mental states via constantly reconstructing a representation of the client's mind and communicating it back to the client. The enhancement of the client's mentalising capacity relies on the therapist drawing attention to the client's internal states inviting the client to explore them further via asking questions, offering alternative perspectives, and reflecting on the affect in the therapeutic relationship (Allen & Fonagy, 2006).

Interestingly, with the exception of Eric's dream interpretation in the first subtheme, participants in this study did not recall any other key interpretations that led to significant transformations/insight. Instead, they focused more on the process of client–therapist interaction as transformative. Thus the process of therapeutic action as painted by the participants here is not in line with traditional psychoanalytic theories which paid more attention to how the unconscious becomes conscious via insightful interpretations, mainly of transference, delivered by therapists who hold the knowledge (Bibring, 1954; Freud, 1916–1917) and reconstruction of repressed infantile memories (Blum, 2003). This is not surprising, as DIT does not prioritise interpretations over other techniques not traditionally seen as active ingredients of change, such as questions, clarification and reflection (Lemma, Target, & Fonagy, 2011), favouring the emergence of preconscious material collaboratively re-examined through the therapist's eyes. It is this process itself, which also maps on to the concept of mentalisation (Allen & Fonagy, 2006) that is viewed as transformative. This conclusion echoes Fonagy's (2003) idea of reconstruction of memories not being an essential change mechanism in psychodynamic therapy, as expressed in his debate with Blum (2003). Other qualitative studies (Lilliengren & Werbart, 2005; Midgley et al., 2006) investigating clients' experiences of other forms of psychodynamic psychotherapy have drawn similar conclusions, emphasising the role of the therapeutic relationship itself and the engagement in reflective thinking over the role of interpretations in the process of therapeutic change. However, the retrospective nature of participants' accounts, which is an inherent limitation of this methodological paradigm as discussed later in this section, may have inadvertently led to such results, as participants are left with a general sense of what was helpful in therapy rather than being able to recall specific events.

Overall participants in this study described an interplay between insight-oriented and relational factors underlying the process of therapeutic change, which supports the view that interpretative and interactional mechanisms in psychoanalysis go hand-in-hand with each other (Stern et al., 1998). In fact, Angela referred explicitly to how feelings of safety in the therapeutic relationship were necessary to facilitate an exploration of feelings that she previously denied. This is in line with the idea that the process of mentalisation takes place effectively only in the context of secure attachment relationships (Fonagy et al., 2002).

The active ingredients of DIT reported by the participants in this study mostly overlap with the theoretical ideas and techniques emphasised by the DIT model. In particular, DIT places the formulation of the IPAF, which allows clients to conceptualise their problems in emotional and interpersonal terms, and the process of mentalisation at the core of the model. It also clearly acknowledges the central role of the therapeutic relationship, the relevance of the concept of attachments and the value of working in the transference, which are all used to support the exploration of the focal pattern (Lemma et al., 2011). The model gives less theoretical emphasis on the development of a coherent narrative, described in the final subtheme, as a vehicle of change. Yes, this process may be implicitly reflected in the central role of the construction of IPAF, which is effectively a short hand narrative reconstructing developmental models and linking them to present day relationships throughout therapy.

A relevant question is to what extent the processes of change that were reported by the participants here are unique to DIT and psychodynamic psychotherapy in general. Unfortunately, without a comparison group, it is difficult to draw definite conclusions about this. However, drawing a comparison between the reported active ingredients of DIT here and the elements identified as distinct of psychodynamic therapy in a literature review of processes research (Blagys & Hilsenroth, 2000), many similarities can be noticed. In particular, both the current study and the above review report a focus on affect and interpersonal experiences, identification of patterns, and an emphasis on the therapeutic relationship and the past. Blagys and Hilsenroth (2000) additionally report the exploration of fantasy life and of non-conscious attempts hindering the therapeutic process as distinct elements of psychodynamic therapy, which, however, have not been reported by the participants in this study. This could be attributed to methodological differences between the studies and the semi-structured nature of DIT emphasising certain interventions over other ones. Shedler (2010) discusses how all the above elements may operate as salient active ingredients of therapy in other treatment models, including CBT. Following his line of thinking, one could then tentatively entertain the idea that the mechanics of change identified in DIT in this study may apply beyond this particular model and psychodynamic therapy in general. Such a hypothesis merits further investigation.

Limitations

The above study is a small-scale qualitative study about the active ingredients of DIT from clients' perspectives, as those demonstrated using IPA. The four subthemes emerged suggest a combination of relational and insight-oriented mechanisms taking place in DIT, most of which are predicted by DIT theory about change. The limitations of the current study need to be taken into account when considering the transferability of the above findings. Such limitations include the small sample size and low response rate as well as the retrospective method of recruitment used (see Leonidaki, Lemma, & Hobbis, 2016). Additionally, an inherent limitation of the current study design is that it relies on participants' retrospective recall of therapy, which may distort their memories. Despite these limitations, the richness of the findings provides some novel ideas about the processes of change in DIT, which may help clinicians apply the model more effectively and contribute to the existing literature about the active ingredients of psychodynamic psychotherapy.

Disclosure statement

No potential conflict of interest was reported by the authors.

Note

1. Italics reflect participant's emphasis on these words.

References

Alexander, F., & French, T. M. (1946). *Psychoanalytic therapy*. New York, NY: Ronald Press.

Allen, J. G., & Fonagy, P. (2006). *Handbook of mentalization-based treatment*. Chichester: Wiley.

American Psychiatric Association. (2000). *Diagnostic and statistical manual of mental disorders: Text revision (DSM-IV-TR* (4th ed.). Washington, DC: Author.

American Psychological Association. (2013). Recognition of psychotherapy effectiveness. *Psychotherapy, 50*, 102–109.

Beck, A. T., Rush, J. A., Shaw, B. F., & Emery, G. (1987). *Cognitive therapy for depression*. New York, NY: Guilford Press.

Beutler, L. E., Malik, M., Alimohamed, S., Harwood, T. M., Talebi, H., Noble, S., & Wong, E. (2003). Therapist variables. In M. J. Lambert (Ed.), *Bergin and Garfield's handbook of psychotherapy and behaviour change* (5th ed., pp. 227–306). Chicago, IL: Wiley.

Bibring, E. (1954). Psychoanalysis and the dynamic psychotherapies. *Journal of the American Psychoanalytic Association, 2*, 745–770.

Blagys, M. D., & Hilsenroth, M. J. (2000). Distinctive features of short-term psychodynamic-interpersonal psychotherapy: A review of the comparative psychotherapy process literature. *Clinical Psychology: Science and Practice, 7*(2), 167–188.

Blum, H. (2003). Response to Peter Fonagy. *International Journal of Psychoanalysis, 84*(3), 509–513. doi:10.1516/3GRX-N11K-6EXK-BG7E

Bowins, B. (2004). Psychological defence mechanisms: A new perspective. *The American Journal of Psychoanalysis, 64*(1), 1–26. doi:10.1023/B:TAJP.0000017989.72521.26

Bowlby, J. (1969/1982). Attachment and loss: Vol. 1. Attachment. New York, NY: Basic Books.

Bowlby, J. (1973). *Attachment and loss, Vol. 2: Separation.* New York, NY: Basic Books.

Bowlby, J. (1988). *A secure base: Parent-child attachment and healthy human development*. New York, NY: Basic Books.

Burns, D., & Nolen-Hoeksema, S. (1992). Therapeutic empathy and recovery from depression in cognitive-behavioral therapy: A structural equation model. *Journal of Consulting and Clinical Psychology, 60*, 441–449.

Department of Health. (2008). *Improving access to psychological therapies: Commissioning for the whole community*. London: Author. Retrieved from http://www.dh.gov.uk/health/category/publications

Department of Health. (2010). *Equity and excellence: Liberating the NHS*. London: Author.

Elliott, R. (2010). Psychotherapy change process research: Realizing the promise. *Psychotherapy Research, 20*(2), 123–135. doi:10.1080/10503300903470743

Fonagy, P. (2003). Rejoinder to Harold Blum. *International Journal of Psychoanalysis, 84*(3), 503–509. doi:10.1516/RHV1-L7KE-G18B-VY6C

Fonagy, P. (2010). Psychotherapy research: Do we know what works for whom? *The British Journal of Psychiatry, 197*, 83–85. doi: 10.1192/bjp.bp.110.079657.Fonagy

Fonagy, P., Gergely, G., Jurist, G., & Target, M. (2002). *Affect regulation, mentalization and the development of the self.* London: Karnac Books.

Freud, S. (1916–1917/1961). Introductory lectures on psycho-analysis Parts I, II, and III. In J. Strachey (Ed. and Trans.). *The standard edition of the complete psychological works of Sigmund Freud* (Vol 15 and 16, pp 1–244). London: Hogarth Press.

Glickauf-Hughes, C., & Wells, M. (1997). *Object relations psychotherapy: An individualized and interactive approach to diagnosis and treatment*. London: Karnac Books.

Grencavage, L. M., & Norcross, J. C. (1990). Where are the commonalities among the therapeutic common factors? *Professional Psychology: Research and Practice, 21*, 372–378.

Hamill, M., Ried, M., & Reynolds, S. (2008). Letters in cognitive analytic therapy: The patients experience. *Psychotherapy Research, 18*(5), 573–583.

Holmes, J. (2002). *The search for the secure base: Attachment theory and psychotherapy*. Guilford: Taylor and Francis.

Horvath, A. O. (2006). The alliance in context: Accomplishments, challenges, and future directions. *Psychotherapy: Theory, Research, Practice, Training, 43*(3), 258–263. doi:10.1037/0033-3204.43.3.258

Ingram, R. E., & Luxton, D. (2005). Vulnerability-stress models. In B. L. Hankin & J. R. Z. Abela (Eds.), *Development of psychopathology: A vulnerability-stress perspective* (pp. 32–46). New York, NY: Sage.

Kernberg, O. F. (2007). The therapeutic action of psychoanalysis: Controversies and challenges. *Psychoanalytic Quarterly, 93*(2), 427–442. doi:10.1111/j.1745-8315.2011.00512.x

Kopta, S. M., Lueger, R. J., Saunders, S. M., & Howard, K. (1999). Individual psychotherapy outcome and process research: Challenges leading to greater turmoil or a positive transition? *Annual Review of Psychology, 50*, 441–469.

Lambert, M. J. (1992). Psychotherapy outcome research: Implications for integrative and eclectic therapists. In J. C. Norcross & M. R. Goldfried (Eds.), *Handbook of psychotherapy integration* (pp. 94–129). New York, NY: Basic.

Lambert, M. J. (2013). The efficacy and effectiveness of psychotherapy. In M. J. Lambert (Ed.), *Bergin and Garfield's handbook of psychotherapy and behavior change* (6th ed.). (pp. 169–218). Hoboken, NJ: Wiley.

Larkin, M., Watts, S., & Clifton, E. (2006). Giving voice and making sense in interpretative phenomenological analysis. *Qualitative Research in Psychology, 3*, 102–120. doi:10.1191/1478088706qp062oa

Lemma, A., Roth, A., Pilling, S. (2008). *The competences required to deliver effective psychoanalytic/psychodynamic therapy*. London: HMSO, Department of Health. Retrieved from www.ucl.ac.uk/CORE

Lemma, A., Target, M., & Fonagy, P. (2010). The development of a brief psychodynamic protocol for depression: Dynamic Interpersonal Therapy (DIT). *Psychoanalytic Psychotherapy, 24*(4), 329–346. doi:10.1521/psyc.2011.74.1.41

Lemma, A., Target, M., & Fonagy, P. (2011). *Brief dynamic interpersonal therapy: A clinician's guide*. Oxford: Oxford University Press.

Leonidaki, V., Lemma, A., & Hobbis, I. (2016). Clients' experiences of dynamic interpersonal therapy (DIT): Opportunities and challenges for brief, manualised psychodynamic therapy in the NHS. *Psychoanalytic Psychotherapy, 30*(1), 42–61.

Lilliengren, P. (2014). *Exploring therapeutic action in psychoanalytic psychotherapy: Attachment to therapist and change*. Stockholm: Department of Psychology, Stockholm University.

Lilliengren, P., & Werbart, A. (2005). A model of therapeutic action grounded in the patients' view of curative and hindering factors in psychoanalytic psychotherapy. *Psychotherapy: Theory, Research, Practice, Training, 42*(3), 324–339. doi:10.1037/a0021179

Martin, D. J., Garske, J. P., & Davis, M. K. (2000). Relation of the therapeutic alliance with outcome and other variables: A meta analytic review. *Journal of Consulting and Clinical Psychology, 68*, 438–450. doi:10.1037/0022-006X.68.3.438

Midgley, N., Target, M., & Smith, J. (2006). The outcome of child psychoanalysis from the patient's point of view: A qualitative analysis of a long-term follow-up study. *Psychology and Psychotherapy: Theory, Research and Practice, 79*, 257–269.
Phillips, J. (1999). The psychodynamic narrative. In G. Roberts & J. Holmes (Eds.), *Healing stories: Narrative in psychiatry and psychotherapy* (pp. 27–49). Oxford: Oxford University Press.
Roth, A., & Fonagy, P. (2005). *What works for whom? A critical review of psychotherapy research.* New York, NY: The Guilford Press.
Schwaber, E. A. (1996). Towards a definition of the term and concept of interaction: Its reflection in analytic listening. *Psychoanalytic Inquiry, 16*(1), 5–24.
Shedler, J. (2010). The efficacy of psychodynamic psychotherapy. *American Psychologist, 65*(2), 98–109. doi:10.1037/a0018378
Smith, M. L., Glass, G. V., & Miller, T. I. (1980). *The benefits of psychotherapy*. Baltimore, Md: Johns Hopkins University Press.
Stern, D. N., Sander, L. W., Nahum, J. P., Harrison, A. M., Lyons-Ruth, K., Morgan, A. C., ... Tronick, E. Z. (1998). Non-interpretive mechanisms in psychoanalytic therapy, the 'something more' than interpretation. The process of change study group. *The International Journal of Psychoanalysis, 79*(5), 903–921.
Sullivan, H. S. (1953). *The interpersonal theory of psychiatry*. New York, NY: Norton.
Todd, D. M., Deane, F. P., & Bragdon, R. A. (2003). Client and therapist reasons for termination: A conceptualisation and preliminary validation. *Journal of Clinical Psychology, 59*(1), 133–147.
Westen, D. (1988). Transference and information processing. *Clinical Psychology Review, 8*(2), 161–179.
World Health Organisation. (1992). *ICD-10 classifications of mental and behavioural disorder: Clinical descriptions and diagnostic guidelines*. Geneva: Author.
Yakeley, J., & Wood, H. (2011). Patients' experiences of forensic psychotherapy. *Psychoanalytic Psychotherapy, 25*(1), 105–114. doi:10.1080/02668734.2010.519160

The process of change in ethnic minority males undergoing psychodynamic psychotherapy: a detailed comparison of two cases

Tohar Dolev, Sigal Zilcha-Mano, Harold Chui, Marna S. Barrett, Kevin S. McCarthy and Jacques P. Barber

Better understanding of the connection between therapeutic processes and outcomes in minority groups can help design and use culturally adapted treatments. To explore the active ingredient in the therapeutic process, the present case study compared two ethnic minority male clients, recruited as part of a randomized controlled trial, one with a good outcome, the other with a poor one. The 12-item Working Alliance Inventory-Observer (S-WAI-O) coding system was used to capture the process of change, alongside a qualitative analysis of content. The cases were identified based on their change in pre- to post-treatment scores on the Beck Depression Inventory and the Hamilton Rating Scale for Depression. The findings suggest a rupture-resolution process in the good outcome case, including a process of negotiation of the alliance and work on issues of trust. In contrast, the poor outcome case showed strong and steady alliance, but context analysis pointed to withdrawal ruptures. Although it is difficult to generalize from a two-case study analysis, the present work suggests that building and negotiating alliance with minority clients has a potential for treatment success.

Most of alliance research to date has not focused on minority clients. Therefore, more research is needed to examine the relationship between minority status and alliance (Castonguay, Constantino, & Holtforth, 2006). Freud was first to discuss the therapeutic relationships, in his early papers on transference (Freud, 1920). Emphasizing the importance of the personal bond between client and therapist, he noted that these bonds help clients remain in therapy and effectively participate in it. The term 'alliance' was later coined by Zetzel (1956) and elaborated by Greenson (1965). Subsequently, Bordin (1979) developed the working alliance framework, suggesting that an effective and positive alliance between clients and therapists comprises three components: the emotional bond within the therapeutic dyad, agreement on the goals of therapy, and agreement on the tasks involved in achieving these goals. Over the years, the topic of therapeutic alliance has received a great deal of attention. Researchers commonly recognize that stronger therapeutic alliance correlates positively with greater symptomatic changes (Martin, Garske, & Davis, 2000). Furthermore, meta-analyses have shown that therapeutic alliance is a predictor of positive outcome in therapy, regardless of differences in treatment conditions (Horvath, Del Re, Flückiger, & Symonds, 2011).

The client–therapist alliance has been noted to be a dynamic construct (de Roten et al., 2004; Stiles & Goldsmith, 2010). Several distinct patterns of alliance development, associated with positive outcomes, have been identified (Stiles & Goldsmith, 2010). Some studies have shown a linear increase in alliance as therapy progresses (Patton, Kivlighan, & Multon, 1997), whereas others have shown a U-shaped pattern (strong alliance in early sessions, decrease during intermediate sessions, and strong alliance in the concluding sessions) and patterns of alliance ruptures and repairs (Safran & Muran, 1996). When predicting positive outcome alliance patterns were found to vary, and to be affected by the rater, whether it was client or therapist rated (Bachelor, 2013). This leaves open the question whether different clients or groups of clients are associated with different and distinct patterns of alliance in successful treatments. In particular, the relationship between therapeutic alliance and symptom change is less clear regarding members of minority groups, where fewer studies have been conducted. Adapting treatment to individual clients has been slower than expected because not enough is known about various groups of clients (Hall, 2001). Several studies have suggested that minorities and non-minorities experience similar benefits from therapy (Blom et al., 2010; Cruz et al., 2007; Lambert et al., 2006), with mixed results in the outcome with mixed and same-race dyads (Imel et al., 2011; Karlsson, 2005). This further underlines the need to examine the processes involved in therapy involving ethnic minority clients.

Of the few studies that have examined differences in therapeutic processes with ethnic minority clients, some discuss the changes that need to be made to the therapeutic process to achieve culturally competent psychotherapy (Bernal, Jiménez-Chafey, & Domenech Rodríguez, 2009; Gaztambide, 2012). Cultural skepticism has been used as a perspective in examining therapeutic sessions (Earl, Alegría, Mendieta, & Linhart, 2011). For example, African Americans have been found to harbor cultural distrust of the psychological field, which may account for an often-noted hesitation to seek treatment, and for the difficulties encountered in it (Brown, Blackmon, & Schumacher, 2013). Racial aspects are present in many treatments, but whether or not they are specifically addressed in therapy does not predict client satisfaction. It has been argued that a humble, empathic, and non-judgmental response from the therapist is of great importance for the success of treatment of ethnic minorities (Chang & Berk, 2009; Owen et al., 2015). In a meta-analysis, therapists' multicultural competence was found to be positively associated with the working alliance (Tao, Owen, Pace, & Imel, 2015). Therefore, it has been argued that it is crucial to adapt psychotherapy to minorities for it to be successful (Pieterse, Todd, Neville, & Carter, 2012).

Consistent with general alliance research, good alliance with minority clients appears to be associated with better outcomes and with higher rates of treatment completion (Cordaro, Tubman, Wagner, & Morris, 2012). Only a few studies, however, have examined the association between alliance, ethnicity, and treatment outcomes in minorities, and these yielded mixed results. For example, some did not find any differences in alliance rating between mixed and same ethnic dyads (Cruz et al., 2007), whereas others found higher therapist- and client-rated alliance, and better outcome in same than in mixed ethnic dyads (Wintersteen, Mensinger, & Diamond, 2005). In a study examining changes in alliance over time, white clients reported a linear increase in alliance over time, whereas ethnic minorities showed no significant changes (Walling, Suvak, Howard, Taft, & Murphy, 2012).

The alliance might be experienced differently by ethnic minority clients, and may inhibit negative reactions toward others, specifically toward the therapist (Vasquez, 2007). A study that examined therapeutic alliance in the treatment of ethnic minorities stressed the importance of addressing the ethnic component and attempting to bridge the ethnic gap (Chang & Berk, 2009). Similar findings were reported in a case study analysis (Knight, 2013). It has been further found that clients who perceived microaggression (subtle forms of racism; Sue et al., 2007) during treatment reported a lower alliance, suggesting that it is important to explore and discuss cultural aspects in treatment and attend to the therapeutic relationship (Owen et al., 2011). To achieve a better understanding of such aspects, it is critical to investigate the therapeutic alliance in individual case studies involving minority clients, which can shed light on the unique processes taking place in the alliance, and on the effect of such processes on treatment outcome. In a case example, Altman (1995) examined how his own feelings of shame as a therapist treating an African American man held him back from bringing up racial content.

In light of the sparse literature on therapeutic alliance with minority clients and of the many open questions that remain in this field, the present study examined the active ingredients in therapeutic process involving minority clients in two cases, one with a good, the other with a poor outcome. We sought to identify the individual-level processes that led to the therapeutic change, and to examine the effect of addressing cultural aspects in treatment. The literature stresses the importance of addressing race-related content and of building trust, but it has not focused specifically on the effect of the dynamic of alliance on outcome involving ethnic minorities. In the present study, we hypothesize that the relationship between the ethnicity of the client and therapist may facilitate racial processes that may need to be carefully attended to. Case study methodology offers an excellent opportunity to investigate mechanisms of change in individual client–therapist dyads and to isolate the mechanisms of change (Hill, Carter, & O'Farrell, 1983). Whereas in large samples researchers can generalize their findings, in case studies it is possible to look deeper into the individual clients and specific changes, enabling the findings to inspire future research of large samples. Use of similar cases treated by the same therapist provides an opportunity to focus on the client and on dyadic variables rather than on the therapist (O'Farrell, Hill, & Patton, 1986).

The two cases reported in the present study were selected from a larger randomized controlled trial (RCT) of short-term psychodynamic psychotherapy, medication, and pill placebo, conducted on 156 clients with major depression disorder (MDD) (Barber, Barrett, Gallop, Rynn, & Rickels, 2012). The RCT found that race and gender moderated outcome. Psychotherapy was found to be more efficacious for minority men than medication and pill placebo. These findings led to the present study, in which we looked deeper into the treatment of this subpopulation to find the active ingredient in psychotherapy that led to the efficacious outcome among minority men. We used a mixed method approach of inquiry that combines qualitative and quantitative tools, one method shedding light on the other to advance clinical knowledge (Dattilio, Edwards, & Fishman, 2010).

Method

The present study relied on an RCT conducted by Barber et al. (2012), in which 156 clients, who had all met the DSM-IV criteria for MDD based on the Structured Clinical Interview (First, Spitzer, Gibbon, & Williams, 1995), were randomized into one of three treatment groups: supportive-expressive therapy (SET), pharmacotherapy, or pill placebo. The clients signed a consent form allowing videotapes of their sessions to be used for research, and were assured that no identification information would be included in any publication. For the purpose of the present study, the therapies of two ethnic-minority males were compared. The clients who were selected had completed the full active phase of SET treatment in the above-mentioned study and had been treated by the same therapist, so that the focus of the study was on clients and dyads rather than on therapists. From among the clients with the most extensive and available record of therapy sessions, two clients were chosen. A single client with the best outcome was selected, he was then matched, based on intake Beck Depression Inventory (BDI) scores and demographic similarities, with a poor outcome case treated by the same therapist. Good and poor outcome cases were identified based on their change in pre- to post-treatment scores on the BDI and the HRSD.

Participants

Client 1

An African-American male in his late thirties, single, father of two children from two women, with 13 years of education, a full-time position in the field of finance, and a moderate annual salary (median, according to the US Census; Webster & Bishaw, 2007). The client claimed that he had been in a depressed state for a few years, which had affected him both socially and professionally. In particular, he noted that his work capacity and professional involvement had decreased, affecting his salary, and that in recent years he had become less active and more withdrawn socially. He sought therapy to address this long-term depressive condition.

Client 2

An African-American male in his late forties, married, father to one child, with 10 years of education, previously employed as a service provider, but unemployed at the time of the study. While employed, the client's annual income had been below the median (according to the US Census; Webster & Bishaw, 2007). The client described a variety of social and mental problems he had faced in the last few years. He felt that he had become withdrawn from his family and friends, that he was not contributing as much as he would have liked to them, and was not as involved as he would have liked to be in the relationships with them. He had sought therapy to address this long-term depressive state.

Therapist

A white female, with over 15 years of clinical experience and over 10 years of experience in SET, who served as a therapist in prior SET studies.

Treatment

Both clients were treated with SET – a time-limited, manualized psychodynamic treatment adapted for depression, using supportive and expressive components (Luborsky et al., 1995). The active treatment lasted 16 weeks. Therapy sessions were provided twice a week during the first four weeks (for a total of 8 sessions), and weekly for the remainder of the treatment, consistent with the process described by Barber et al. (2012). The treatment focused on understanding the clients' negative relationship patterns and helping them cope with core relational difficulties, with the use of supportive techniques aimed at establishing positive relationships (Luborsky, 1984). Expressiveness refers to the therapist using that which is expressed by the client to frame interpretations of the main relationship themes. Clinical formulation was based on the Core Conflictual Relationship Theme (CCRT), a method that comprises three components: a wish (W), a response from the other (RO), and a response from the self (RS). CCRT helps track the clients' experiences and can be used to direct therapy sessions to focus on the wishes and hopes of clients within the context of therapy (Luborsky et al., 1995). The treatment manual emphasizes the importance of transference and countertransference work. It has been suggested that therapists should explore cultural issues that may affect the therapeutic work in SET and other psychodynamic treatments (Leichsenring & Schaunburg, 2014); that therapists should be aware of their own and their clients' cultural background and explore the differences between them; and that they should make an effort to become familiar with their client's cultural background, and distinguish between what is normal and what is perceived as impaired in the client's cultural context (Connolly Gibbons et al., 2012).

Measures

The measures of the RCT used in the present study were the BDI (Beck, Ward, & Mendelson, 1961), the Hamilton Rating Scale for Depression (HRSD) (Hamilton, 1960), the Inventory of Interpersonal Problems-Circumplex (IIP-C) (Alden, Wiggins, & Pincus, 1990; Horowitz, Rosenberg, Baer, Ureño, & Villaseñor, 1988), and the Working Alliance Inventory-Short Form: Client and Therapist versions (WAI) (Horvath & Greenberg, 1989) (described in detail in Table 1).

Two further measures were the Segmented Working Alliance Inventory Observer form, and the qualitative analysis of content, described below.

Segmented Working Alliance Inventory Observer form (S-WAI-O) (Berk, 2013)

A 12-item observer-scored inventory, based on Bordin's (1979) conceptualization of the working alliance, consisting of three subscales: bond, task, and goal. In the S-WAI-O only two of the subscales were used: bond and task. The goal subscale was removed because of high correlations and an overlap between the goal and the task items (Berk, 2013). The score is calculated as an average for each subscale, and an overall score for each 5-min segment, measuring change in the quality of the working alliance throughout the therapy session. Higher scores indicate a stronger alliance; a dip or a decline in the alliance rating is considered a rupture. In the present study, two undergraduate students served as independent observers and received training for two intensive weeks, 64 h in total, until agreement between them was achieved. Thirty-four videotaped therapy sessions and 300 segments were coded and analyzed. Inter-judge reliability by the two coders, as assessed by intraclass correlation (ICC [2, 1]; Shrout & Fleiss, 1979), was .93.

Qualitative analysis of content (Braun & Clarke, 2006)

Four researchers analyzed all the therapy sessions of both cases; two of the four researchers were more closely involved in the analysis than the others. Analysis was based on watching the videotaped sessions and looking for interpersonal interactions in the treatment. The aim was to explore the processes taking place in interpersonal interactions between the therapist and the client in the therapy room. The clinical formulation of the treatment (CCRT) was used to identify the patterns of recurrent themes and interpersonal problems in the thematic analysis. We focused on the client's interpersonal patterns and the ways they were or

Table 1. Measures used in the current study.

Measure	Description	Time of assessment in current study
Beck Depression Inventory (BDI) (Beck et al., 1961)	A 21 item self-reported inventory assessing the severity of depression. Higher scores indicate more severe depression	Intake and final session
Hamilton Rating Scale for Depression (HRSD) (Hamilton, 1960)	A 17 item Clinician-based evaluation of depressive symptoms. Higher scores indicate more severe depression	Intake and final session
Inventory of Interpersonal Problems-Circumplex (IIP-C) (Alden et al., 1990; Horowitz et al., 1988)	A 64-item self-reported inventory assessing behaviors related to interpersonal problems. Clients are assigned an overall score indicating their angle with respect to the circumplex as well as a score for each of the eight octants (domineering, vindictive, cold, socially avoidant, nonassertive, exploitable, overly nurturant, and intrusive)	Intake, week eight and final session
Working Alliance Inventory-Short Form: Client and Therapist versions (WAI) (Horvath & Greenberg, 1989)	A 12-item self-reported inventory based on Bordin's (1979) conceptualization of the working alliance. Higher scores indicate stronger alliances	Week two, four, eight, and final session

were not repeated in the interaction with the therapist, in light of the theoretical and empirical expectation that the client's interpersonal problems and interactions are important in maintenance and persistence of depression (Luborsky & Mark, 1991). The detailed analysis enabled us to become familiar with the narrative and the themes in each treatment, provided a better understanding of the therapy process, and led to the identification of unique phases of treatment for each client. Based on these phases, we segmented the treatments into three periods, each period consisting of different processes and themes, to better investigate the various processes.

Results

Client 1: the good outcome case

Background

At intake, the client was found to have moderate-to-severe depression (BDI: 31, and HRSD: 16). The client met criteria for personality disorder not otherwise specified, with narcissistic, borderline, and depressive tendencies. The client did not present comorbidity with any DSM-IV-Axis I anxiety disorders. Based on self-report questionnaires at intake, the client showed high interpersonal distress (IIP-64: 0.80 SD above the norm), in particular, a tendency to be cold or distant in interpersonal relationships, and difficulties in maintaining long-term interpersonal relationships. The client also reported a need to be in control (IIP Angle: 173.38).

Course of treatment

The client's therapy process was divided into three phases: initial, intermediate, and concluding. The decision which sessions were included in each phase was determined based on changes in processes, patterns, and themes, as identified in the coding of the S-WAI-O data (Figure 1(a)). The changes in alliance coding were consistent with the qualitative analysis of content identification of different processes and themes for each phase.

The initial phase consisted of the first six sessions, in which the client described his main interpersonal problems with his mother, with the mother of his son, and with one of his friends. Issues of trust, disrespect, and betrayal were evident. The first source of difficulties in interpersonal relationships to be reported, and the most dominant, had to do with the client's mother. The client noted his disappointment with the way his mother had raised him. Because he would often be left with other family members, he felt neglected. The client described an incident of feeling mistreated and underappreciated when his mother had forgotten to pick him up from school: 'I waited for 13 hours because my mom didn't come to pick me up.' The therapist's response communicated to the client that he should feel free to share his feelings with her, that she had understood his feelings and

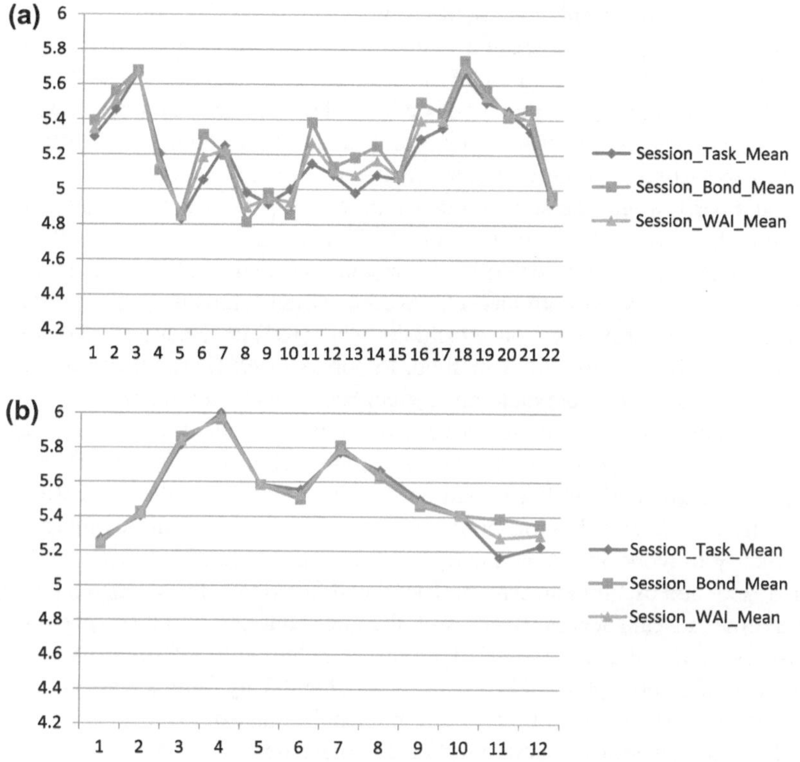

Figure 1. Changes in the ranking of observer coded alliance throughout the therapy sessions. Higher scores indicate a stronger alliance in each of the components of the alliance (task, bond, overall alliance score). Values for 5-min segments were averaged to yield a single score per session. (a) Changes in observer coded alliance values for the 22 sessions of the good outcome case. (b) Changes in observer coded alliance values for the 12 sessions of the poor outcome case.

was supportive of him and critical of the mother for having let him wait for many hours. Following this session, the client's self-reported WAI scores showed that his alliance with the therapist had significantly improved, from WAI: 4.58 at the time of intake, when alliance expectation was lowest, to WAI: 5.41 at the end of the second week of therapy. As is often the case, the therapist's self-reported WAI was lower than the client's WAI (week 2, WAI: 4.25).

Another source of interpersonal problems mentioned by the client in the course of the initial sessions was the mother of his son, to whom he attributed feelings of rejection and disrespect toward him. According to the client, at the beginning of his relationship with his son's mother he had failed to appreciate the relationship they had, and had seen it as temporary. When he realized that he wanted to be with her, she had already 'moved on' and had rejected him. The client voiced many complaints about the way she was raising their son. The client's manner of speech suggested that he might be masking feelings of rejection with complaints about money (for instance, such feelings became apparent when the client complained that when he did not give their son money, the mother would become angry, reject him, and speak ill of him to their son). Further evidence of the sense of being underappreciated emerged when the client described being at a party where the son's mother ignored his presence. He noted a similar pattern with reference to another woman he had dated. In this case, too, the client reported that he had felt rejected by the woman once she realized that he did not have enough money. In both cases, as well as when referring to his mother, the client expressed a strong response from the other (RO) of rejection and disrespect (as conceptualized in the CCRT method, Luborsky (1995)). The therapist showed empathy, and tried to understand and reflect back the client's feelings.

Other than references to the above two women, the client also referred to one of his male friends as disrespectful and as a source of disappointment. He recalled a period when he and the friend had been writing songs together, and was upset by the friend's later behavior, noting that the friend had taken advantage of an opportunity to work on his own and to become successful. The client felt he had been abandoned by him and that the friend had failed to acknowledge the client's part in this musical success. As a result, the client felt hurt and disrespected.

Issues concerning the client's feelings of belonging to a minority came up throughout the initial phase. The client spoke of authority figures who, he felt, had harassed him or had made him feel incompetent because of his race. For example, the client described a previous workplace where he had been late to work and was subsequently fired. He noted that he could not understand the reason for his dismissal and blamed his former boss of racism. Although race-related considerations may indeed have led to his dismissal, and although the client's on-the-job actions may have stemmed from a race-related need to manage his self-esteem defensively, the client directed his anger exclusively at what he viewed as a racist action, and was unable to see any alternative reasons for his dismissal, even with the therapist's guidance.

As a consequence of the above-cited relationship representations, the client initially expressed a strong aversion to needing others. He cited his need for independence as the reason behind his current preference for being self-employed. In the course of the initial therapy sessions, the client came to understand that he had arranged his life in a way that minimized his need for others. However, the client did acknowledge needing his son, and noted that he felt betrayed when the son would not visit him or call him on Fathers' Day. His daughter was not mentioned in this context.

The second phase comprised nine sessions, during which the issue of intimacy emerged. Three themes related to intimacy became evident: the client's need for intimacy with others; the challenges of developing intimacy with the therapist; and, as a result of these challenges, ruptures in the alliance with the therapist (deterioration in the alliance or tension between the client and the therapist

(Safran & Muran, 2006)). During these sessions, a reduction in the client's IIP dominance score (week 8, DOM octant of the IIP: 0.02) indicated that the client had become less domineering.

The client seemed slow to warm up in the interaction with the therapist, and had a difficult time starting almost all sessions, as reflected in the low observer-rated S-WAI-O scores (information obtained from the segmented coding, not the average single session score). It was during these intermediate sessions that the client started to test the client–therapist relationship, questioning the right degree of intimacy for such a bond. The client noted his fear, which may in part have been realistic, of being misunderstood by the therapist. At that point, the client seemed reluctant to open up and talk about relationships with women he was dating, or about issues related to his son. For example, in one of these intermediate sessions, the client commented: 'I have children and we haven't discussed that yet. Hopefully we can avoid that subject for a couple of months.' At the same time, the client expressed the belief and hope that he would be able to open up to the therapist in the future. Later, but during the same phase, when the client was just beginning to open up to the therapist and wanted the therapist to be there for him, he stated: 'I wish I had somebody in my corner.' Similarly, the client's need for greater support from people around him was frustrated by trust issues and by his difficulties in opening up to them, exemplified by his comments about his fear of being used. The client was able to talk about these fears and about his hopes for more intimate relationships. He mentioned several past experiences that highlighted those feelings. In one example, he referred to having 'a yet-undefined relationship' with a woman. In later sessions, during the same intermediate phase, the client realized that he wanted to be with that woman, but after he had approached her, she rejected him. In another instance, the client referred to a woman whom he had been dating and with whom the relationship failed because he felt she had been using him, and had been interested mostly in his money.

As noted above, the intermediate sessions contained many ruptures in the therapeutic relationship. For example, a power-related rupture occurred in week 4, with a meaningful decrease in both bond and task, as demonstrated by S-WAI-O observer coding (Figure 1(a)), with the observer-rated alliance mean reaching its lowest point in the therapy (S-WAI-O: 4.85). This rupture also affected the therapist-reported WAI for the same week (week 4, WAI: 4.17). During this rupture, the client said that he felt it was expected of him to be the first to speak at the opening of the session. He believed that this expectation put him at a disadvantage, as it would, in his opinion, in the case of business relationships. Note that the client was smiling while discussing these feelings, a gesture that may have moderated the effect of his words and provided a sense of hope for the future of their relationship. The therapist responded: 'But we are not in sales, I'm quiet to see where you will pull from.' In an effort to resolve the rupture, the therapist explained the reasons for letting the client speak first, but the client responded that he was not persuaded. Nevertheless, in a subsequent intermediate-phase session, the client no longer viewed himself as inferior to the therapist but rather as an equal contributor to the therapy because he was contributing to research. Additional ruptures with the client had to do with the fact that as he sought respect and equality with the therapist, he had started asking questions about the therapist's personal life, and was trying to mimic the therapist's manner of speaking, saying: 'So, how are you? Did you have a good week?'

Subsequent rupture resolution processes, in which the therapist explicitly addressed the rupture between them, appear to have helped the client open up to the therapist and feel respected. In one example, the therapist inquired whether the client had been abusing drugs: 'Are you on any substances that are making it hard for you?' The client was offended and stated: 'It's possible that I'm like this without chemical use.' However, after the therapist apologized: 'Sorry if I had offended you,' the apology seemed to have a positive effect on the client. The same event also provided an example of a micro-aggression. The client said: 'Well you accused me of being a pot head.' Following this encounter, the atmosphere between the therapist and the client seemed to become more comfortable, with both adopting a more relaxed posture and smiling more frequently at each other.

The means by which the ruptures were resolved, through empathy and openness of the therapist, appeared to promote a facilitating environment, which in turn, allowed the alliance between the client and therapist to grow stronger in the following sessions, as the client started to share and open up more. The therapist accomplished this by choosing not to avoid starting a direct discussion when the client raised racial concerns. This resolution of ruptures was also reflected in the client's reported WAI, which was lower, but still above his average alliance of 5.11 (Week 4: WAI: 5.25). Throughout this phase, the therapist was active, giving concrete advice and using supportive techniques, consistent with the model of SET, and the client appeared to follow her advice. The client also seemed more content with his relationships with his son and family. His depression symptoms were similarly improving, with the lowest score noted for session 15, BDI: 15.

The third phase comprised the last seven therapy sessions, during which the client recognized the work and commitment he had invested in the therapy, in particular with regard to the interpersonal relationship with the therapist: 'I don't think I did anything that required a commitment before this one.' The client attended all sessions and understood their significance. This recognition was further evident in the overall client IIP score, which decreased to its lowest value on week 16 (week 2-IIP: 0.80; week 16-IIP: 0.48). The therapist also praised the client's hard work during the course of the therapy, and demonstrated a high degree of empathy toward him. During this phase, the client felt comfortable discussing his difficulties beyond his financial problems, and was beginning to understand, with the help of the therapist, that his happiness was not dependent upon financial success, as he had thought earlier. The client was also able to acknowledge that earning more money would not make him happier and became aware of his need for significant relationships in his life. In particular, he acknowledged that he was looking for more meaningful relationships with women. In another development, the client's son came to visit for the summer, and their relationship became stronger, as they spent more time together and jointly visited the client's family. Congruent with the above findings, the observer WAI scores for this phase showed an increase in both task and bond. The therapist's self-reported WAI also increased, from WAI: 4.25 on week 8 to its highest point, WAI: 4.75, on week 16.

The observer S-WAI-O scores (Figure 1(a)) show a jagged pattern in the last sessions. This occurred simultaneously with an increase in the client's self-reported WAI scores on week 8 (WAI: 5.08) and week 16 (WAI: 5.25). In the final session, however, the client felt that he had not progressed enough, and ruptures appeared, associated with the end of the therapy and the upcoming separation from the therapist and with the confidentiality of the therapy. The therapist tried to reassure the client, and her attempts appeared to be successful.

External observation of alliance (S-WAI-O)

Fluctuations in the observer S-WAI-O, with a significant number of low rupture points, were noted mostly in the intermediate sessions (Figure 1(a)), corresponding to the period when the alliance and the relationship between client and therapist were being negotiated, in particular issues related to trust and self-disclosure.

Self-report data

The self-reported data suggest a process similar to that reflected by the S-WAI-O. Throughout the course of the therapy, both the client's and therapist's self-reported WAI values were moderate (Table 2). Changes in client–therapist alliance rating in the course of the therapy reflected a strengthening of the alliance, with a decrease in week 8 for the client. IIP scores at intake indicated a cold tendency and problems in the areas of trust (vindictive octant of the IIP: 1.19) and of

Table 2. All available client and therapist rated WAI.

Client 1 WAI			Client 2 WAI		
Week	Client self-reported WAI	Therapist self-reported WAI	Week	Client self-reported WAI	Therapist self-reported WAI
Intake	4.58		Intake		
Week 2	5.42	4.25	Week 2		5.25
Week 4	5.25	4.17	Week 4	6.75	
Week 8	5.08	4.25	Week 8	6.58	5.75
Week 16	5.25	4.75	Week 16	6.50	6.00

Note: WAI = working alliance inventory.

the establishment of close relationships with others (cold octant of the IIP: 2.57). In later sessions, a history of being taken advantage of by others was revealed, which had not been referred to in the client's self-report (exploitable octant of the IIP: −1.00). This omission may indicate a need to appear strong and to not need others. Overall angle scores pointed to a cold orientation (173.38), but in the course of therapy a change toward less cold and more vindictive (159.75) was noted. The most significant improvements over the course of the therapy were noted in the domineering and non-assertive octants. Improvement was shown in both BDI and HRSD outcome measures over the course of the treatment. Change was most prominent in the second and third phases of therapy.

Client 2: poor outcome case

Background

At intake, the client was diagnosed with major depressive disorder (BDI: 33 and HRSD: 28, indicating severe depression). The client showed no comorbidity with any Axis-I or personality disorders. Based on the self-report questionnaires at intake, the client showed very high interpersonal distress (IIP-64: 1.26 points above the norm). A cold and social avoidant interpersonal orientation was noted. In particular, he reported being anxious in the presence of others, not initiating social interactions, and lacking self-confidence (Angle: 193.25).

Course of therapy

Similar to the good-outcome case, this client's therapy sessions can be divided into three phases: initial, intermediate, and concluding, based on the identification of different processes, patterns, and themes, as rated on the S-WAI-O (Figure 1(b)). Changes in alliance coding were consistent with the qualitative processes and themes noted for each phase.

The initial phase: The first five sessions were characterized by the client's idealization of his own 'previous self,' before becoming depressed. Two years prior to therapy, he saw himself, as a social person, close to his friends and family, active and respected at work, and always employed in fulfilling jobs. Since then, the client reported that he had been depressed, unable to sleep or to form social interactions. During one of the early therapy sessions, he commented: 'I have been avoiding people for a long time, haven't been socializing at all.' He was unable to identify a specific incident that had led to these feelings of depression and low self-worth. Although acknowledging these feelings to the therapist, the client felt a need to hide them from others. He thought that by acknowledging such feelings he would be letting down his friends and his family. The client also felt that he was not meeting his social obligations, such as playing with his daughter or participating in family events. He noted a particular family event in which he had not wanted to participate so as not to draw attention to his problem, and stated:

'I haven't even told my own people.' The client explained that he avoided social contact because he did not want others to feel sorry for him and because of a need to appear as if he was doing well. The client appeared to try to maintain a sense of self-worth. The therapist was empathic and reported a relatively high WAI at week 2 (WAI: 5.25).

The client's apparent fear to let others down was noted in several of his comments, and was reflected by his high IIP scores at intake (IIP nonassertive octant: 0.85). For example, the client reported that when offered a new employment opportunity, he was afraid to accept it so as not to let the boss down if he turned out to be unable to fulfill the requirements of the position. Another example had to do with his concern about his sexual performance with his wife. Similarly, in the course of the therapy, the client often asked the therapist to reassure him that he was doing a good job. Throughout this phase, the therapist was helpful, reassuring the client and giving him concrete advice, to which the client responded either by nodding or with statements of passive agreement (e.g. 'Yeah, you're right').

The alliance between the client and the therapist appeared to grow as the sessions progressed, as evidenced by an increase in observer S-WAI-O scores, for both task and bond. The client participated actively in the therapy, agreed with the therapist, echoed her words, and seemed to follow all her suggestions. This acceptance may have been the reason for the noted increase in the therapist's WAI scores. Ruptures were not apparent on the surface during the early therapy sessions, but the increase in alliance was not followed by a corresponding improvement in the client's depression symptoms, as evidenced both by his self-report (week 3, BDI: 28) and his restless sleep. The client was still seeking reassurances from the therapist, and would often ask: 'So you think I should do it?'

The second phase consisted of four sessions. Examination of the data recorded at these sessions showed that the client often seemed to agree with the therapist's advice, but later would not act upon it. For example, the therapist advised him to see a specialist for the headaches he had been reporting, and the client agreed to do so, but in the end did not. The same pattern was apparent in the client's relationship with his wife: he promised his wife that he would go with her to church, but failed to do so. In yet another instance, the therapist recommended some nutritious beverages and healthy foods that she thought would improve the clients' appetite and energy levels. After some initial hesitation, the client did try the beverages, but two weeks later he stopped using them. The client's WAI scores during these sessions increased from the expected alliance at intake (WAI: 5.66) to their highest rating in the fourth week (week 4, WAI: 6.75). The S-WAI-O observer graph (Figure 1(b)) shows that the strong alliance with the therapist, noted already in the initial phase of therapy, persisted, but content analysis demonstrated the client's lack of commitment to following the therapist's suggestions. The client may have pretended to accept the therapist's suggestions only to avoid disagreements. The client's self-reported depression symptoms were lowest during these sessions (BDI: 16), although Hamilton scores remained high (HRSD: 27).

One of the themes brought up by the client during this phase was the subject of trust. When, on one occasion, the therapist mentioned having children, the disclosure seemed to please the client, who said: 'It makes me happy to know you have kids,' and appeared to bolster the bond between the two, allowing the client to open up more about his own daughter. Therapist self-disclosure during this phase of therapy may have contributed to a high self-reported WAI scores by the client (week 8, WAI: 6.58) and the therapist (week 8, WAI: 5.75). In another instance, the subject of trust was discussed following the client's visit to his doctor. The client claimed that the doctor was withholding some medical information pertaining to his case, and shared feelings of being mistreated and lied to. The therapist responded with concrete advice, recommending that the client look for a doctor he trusts.

The third phase consisted of the last three therapy sessions. The themes that emerged during these sessions were similar to the ones noted during the second, intermediate phase of therapy. The client stated that the therapist had helped him a great deal, and even revealed that he had been keeping her phone number in his wallet. At the same time, he still felt that he was not helping enough at home and was not being appreciated for the things he was trying to do. In one case, feelings of worthlessness arose again when the client's wife thought that he should not accompany his daughter on a school field trip, and had asked her brother, the daughter's uncle, to do it instead. The client's overall IIP scores decreased during these last sessions to IIP: 0.42 (as compared with IIP: 1.26 at intake).

During this phase, the topic of the final sessions was discussed. The client found it difficult to adjust to the approaching conclusion of the therapy sessions. Asked by the therapist how he felt about ending the therapy, he said that he had no bad feelings about it, 'but I just figured, that for as long as I can just keep seeing somebody, I will get it done.' The client's reaction was passive, but his disappointment was visible. This pattern was also evident in the decrease in the S-WAI-O (Figure 1(b)) scores during the concluding sessions, as well as in the client's self-reported WAI scores, which decreased in week 16 (WAI: 6.50). The therapist self-reported WAI scores increased, and were highest in week 16 (WAI: 6.00).

During the very last therapy session, the client stated that although he had not wanted to attend this session, he also did not want to disappoint the therapist. In this, as well as in other comments, the client's fear of disappointing others and his seeking of therapist's approval emerged as recurring and persisting themes. Neither the therapist nor the client addressed cultural content, the alliance seemed strong on the surface, and they did not actively work on strengthening the alliance.

External observation of alliance (S-WAI-O)

A high, steady alliance, with no apparent ruptures, was noted throughout the entire treatment (Figure 1(b)). External observations suggested less work on issues of trust and on negotiating the client–therapist relationships. The client made no reference to issues of race at any point in the treatment.

Self-report data

Both the client's and the therapist's self-reported data reflected a strong, steady alliance (Table 2), similar to that revealed by the S-W-AI-O scores. In his IIP questionnaire, the client did report difficulties in establishing close relationships with others (cold octant of the IIP: 1.26), and high levels of anxiety in the presence of others (socially avoidant octant of the IIP: 2.18). Although lack of confidence and some self-doubt were also noted (nonassertive octant of the IIP: 0.85), the client did not see himself as easily persuaded by others (exploitable octant of the IIP: 0.18). With respect to this last element, however, some evidence from the therapy sessions suggested otherwise. Evidence from the client's self-reports also suggests a highly apparent need to please others and to win their approval (overly nurturant octant of the IIP: 1.36). A change from a cold and social avoidant orientation in the client's overall IIP scores (193.25) at intake to a more nonassertive and less cold orientation (260.28) at the end of therapy was noted. The most significant improvement in IIP scores was noted for the vindictive octant. Only an insignificant decrease in the client's BDI, and an even smaller one in his HRSD, was noted over the course of treatment, despite the client's statements to the therapist, during the therapy sessions, that he had seen an improvement in his state.

Discussion

The present study compared in detail two cases to explore and identify potential active ingredients that contribute to the outcome of treatment for minority clients, in particular African-American men, in psychodynamic psychotherapy using a mixed model design. All available records from the clients' therapy sessions were coded using the S-WAI-O, taking into consideration the self-reported WAI scores of the clients and the therapist, as well as other client self-report measures (e.g. the IIP). These data were analyzed in conjunction with a qualitative assessment of the content of the therapy sessions. The mixed method approach used in the present study combines self-reported data and clinically administered measures, with qualitative analysis of content making possible an important comparison between different perspectives of the relationship (client, therapist, and observer). This, in turn, enabled us to observe in-depth the narrative of each client and the dynamics of each treatment, and to carry out an integrative comparison of the two clients. Both clients were African-American males of similar age and depression severity at intake. Both were treated by the same therapist, and both reported interpersonal problems and feelings of incompetence in their interpersonal relationships at the beginning of treatment. Both clients showed a decrease in self-reported interpersonal distress at the end of treatment. There is an open question about the degree of conscious change in the clients regarding their interpersonal problems. The results of the current study may indicate what degree of conscious ability is needed to be able to report difficulties. During treatment, the awareness of difficulties may come up and lead the client to rank higher levels of interpersonal difficulties.

We selected the two clients who differed markedly in their BDI and HRSD outcome scores, with improvement on both measures for the good outcome case, and a much smaller decrease in BDI and almost no change in HRSD for the poor outcome case. The clients differed also in their observer-coded alliance, demonstrating fluctuations in the alliance in the good outcome case, and strong and steady alliance in the poor outcome case. Content analysis, however, revealed that the steady alliance in the poor outcome case included withdrawal ruptures. This became noticeable even when the therapist and client appeared to be working together. Although the client appeared to accept the therapists' suggestions, he also tended to withdraw and avoid disagreements in a way that seemed overly deferential (a behavior pattern previously noted by Safran and Muran (2006); see also Eubanks-Carter, Muran, and Safran (2010)).

We found that the good-outcome client had negotiated his interpersonal needs with the therapist, leading to increased self-disclosure and a stronger alliance. They seemed to be working together and the client opened up emotionally to the therapist. In contrast, the poor-outcome client presented a general façade of well-being, refrained from revealing most of his problems, and was unwilling to negotiate his alliance with the therapist, thus not fully addressing his needs and not raising racial issues, which have been found to be important in working with many minority clients (Chang & Berk, 2009). Underneath the good alliance, the client appears not to have felt that he could raise issues of race and reveal his true feelings about the therapist. These findings confirm the important role of the rupture-resolution process in the therapeutic alliance. Ruptures have been defined as a deterioration, or tension in the alliance (Safran & Muran, 2006), and can describe either a major break in therapy or minor tensions between client and therapist (Safran, Muran, & Eubanks-Carter, 2011). Earlier studies have stressed the importance of the rupture-resolution process for therapy outcomes with non-minority clients. Successful resolution of ruptures can contribute to emotional changes during therapy and to better outcomes (see also Eubanks-Carter et al., 2010). Previous studies found significant correlation between rupture-repair episodes and outcomes, and have shown that the presence of such episodes predicted better outcomes (Safran et al., 2011). The present findings suggest that the benefits from rupture-resolution processes apply to minority clients as well.

A rupture-resolution process was evident in the good outcome case, where a negotiation of the alliance and joint work on issues of trust and self-disclosure were noted. The good outcome case also involved ruptures caused by the racial differences between client and therapist, which were then resolved. By contrast, the poor outcome case showed strong alliance during treatment, but at the same time masking unresolved withdrawal ruptures: the client was overly agreeable and made efforts to draw closer to the therapist and seek her approval, but at the same time he concealed certain personal experiences from her.

The present findings are consistent with previous reports on issues of trust in psychotherapy, regardless of other client characteristics, as well as with previous documented cases in which minority clients were reported to show their distrust of psychotherapy (Brown et al., 2013). In the present study, the therapist and the good-outcome client addressed the multicultural component openly and explicitly, attempting to overcome the ethnic gap, which proved beneficial to the formation of a strong and genuine alliance. In previous studies, such a process was found to be an important factor in the negotiation of the therapeutic alliance for minority clients (Chang & Berk, 2009). In the poor outcome case, the topic of race did not come up. We suggest that the development of trust may be jeopardized and fail if conscious and unconscious culturally specific elements are not brought to awareness during psychoanalytic psychotherapy.

One aspect of the present findings is inconsistent with some previous research: a strong and steady alliance has been previously associated with better outcomes in minority clients (Cordaro et al., 2012), in the present study the poor-outcome client showed a high and steady alliance, which may be attributed to the lack of race-related discussion in treatment, whereas the good-outcome client displayed fluctuating alliance levels. Addressing the cultural aspect in the good outcome case appears to have led to the resolution of ruptures, whereas in the poor outcome case the cultural aspect and the withdrawal ruptures were not addressed. The different outcomes of the two cases attest to the importance of addressing ruptures and resolving them in treatment, and of discussing cultural aspects. Not all clients are able to identify and report on ruptures and various cultural characteristics may mask them. If our finding is replicated in a larger sample, therapists treating minority clients may wish to identify and examine subtle nuances in the therapeutic alliance, and negotiate the therapeutic alliance with their clients, showing responsiveness and sensitivity when clients raise racial issues. In turn, such attention and routine monitoring by the therapist may help elucidate the effect of alliance-focused training for therapists on the outcome of treatment.

The current study highlights the importance of trust in relationships between therapists and minority clients, and the need to boost such trust by means of open discussion and alliance negotiation. If the results are replicated in samples of a larger size, they may suggest that therapists should keep in mind that good alliance may mask withdrawal ruptures. Therapists should note that some minority clients may need more open negotiations of trust and higher levels of self-disclosure about race to form genuine alliances. As suggested by the present findings, these could then lead to better outcomes. To examine cultural sensitivity, a comparison of mixed and non-mixed dyads may be needed. Note, however, that the findings of the present study are consistent with the literature on mixed dyads, showing that the alliance did not increase linearly (Walling et al., 2012).

Limitations

In a case study many factors may be examined, each one leading to a different analysis of the findings. The present study focused mainly on client–therapist alliance as an active ingredient in the therapy. The research data, however, may also be examined from other perspectives. For example, it is possible to examine the therapy processes presented here and the corresponding outcomes from the perspective of the CCRT method, arguing that in the good outcome case CCRT had been formulated and negotiated with the client, whereas in the poor outcome case these steps were less evident for the poor outcome client. Other therapy approaches may have treated race and culture differently leading to different outcomes. Additional perspectives on the two cases may also look into the coding of culture processes of the clients in relation to outcome, exploring macro-aggression and cultural identity. Examining the alliance from multiple perspectives, based on client and therapist self-reports and on observer coding, can shed light on the therapy process. The design of the present study, however, leaves the important question of causality unanswered. Future studies are needed, using the hermeneutic single-case efficacy design (HSCED, Elliott, 2002), which can be useful in evaluating treatment causality in single therapy cases, especially to establish a causal link between the therapy process and outcome.

The two clients presented in this study differed from one another in many ways, including marital status and income, and these differences may have contributed to differences in their behavior and in the outcomes. The clients differed from the therapist in gender and ethnicity, whereas matched therapist–client dyads may lead to different outcomes. This limitation, however, is mitigated by the fact that in our study the therapist was the same in both cases, and their pretreatment depression symptoms were matched. In larger sample sizes, it is also important to disentangle differences between clients based on trait-like characteristics (such as the baseline differences in symptomatology and comorbidity between cases) and the effect of the dynamic nature of the alliance within each client, such as rupture and repair processes (Zilcha-Mano, 2017). Such analyses will help better identify dynamic processes in the alliance. In addition, conscious and unconscious processes relating to cultures play an important role in therapy, and this separation should be explored in future studies. Finally, we are not able to explain some of the findings, such as the decrease in IIP in both clients; examining other characteristics might elucidate these findings, and using a clinical interview about interpersonal problems may bring up difficulties of which the client is not aware.

Conclusion

Based on two case studies, the present research adds to the growing knowledge regarding alliance with minority clients. Although it is difficult to generalize based on the analysis of two case studies, the present work draws attention to the importance of negotiating both the alliance and other aspects of the relationship between black clients and white therapists, for the success of the treatment.

Disclosure statement

No potential conflict of interest was reported by the authors.

Funding

Written with support from NIMH [grant R01 MH 06141] (Jacques P. Barber, PI). The sponsor did not have any role in the study besides funding the study.

References

Altman, N. (1995). *The Analyst in the inner city: Race, class, and culture through a psychoanalytic lens*. Hillsdale, NJ: The Analytic Press.

Alden, L. E., Wiggins, J. S., & Pincus, A. L. (1990). Construction of circumplex scales for the inventory of interpersonal problems. *Journal of Personality Assessment, 55*, 521–536. doi:10.1207/s15327752jpa5503&410

Bachelor, A. (2013). Clients' and therapists' views of the therapeutic alliance: Similarities, differences and relationship to therapy outcome. *Clinical Psychology & Psychotherapy, 20*, 118–135. doi:10.1002/cpp.792

Barber, J. P., Barrett, M. S., Gallop, R., Rynn, M. A., & Rickels, K. (2012). Short-term dynamic psychotherapy versus pharmacotherapy for major depressive disorder: A randomized, placebo-controlled trial. *The Journal of Clinical Psychiatry, 73*, 66–73. doi:10.4088/JCP.11m06831

Beck, A. T., Ward, C., & Mendelson, M. (1961). Beck depression inventory (BDI). *Achieves of General Psychiatry, 4*, 561–571. doi:10.1037/t00741-000

Berk, E. (2013). *Detecting alliance ruptures and rupture repair with the Segmented Working Alliance Inventory – Observer Form (S-WAI-O)* (Unpublished dissertation). New York, NY: The New School for Social Research.

Bernal, G., Jiménez-Chafey, M. I., & Domenech Rodríguez, M. M. (2009). Cultural adaptation of treatments: A resource for considering culture in evidence-based practice. *Professional Psychology: Research and Practice, 40*, 361–368. doi:10.1037/a0016401

Blom, M. B., Hoek, H. W., Spinhoven, P., Hoencamp, E., Haffmans, P. J., & van Dyck, R. (2010). Treatment of depression in patients from ethnic minority groups in the Netherlands. *Transcultural Psychiatry, 47*, 473–490. doi:10.1177/1363461510374561

Bordin, E. S. (1979). The generalizability of the psychoanalytic concept of the working alliance. *Psychotherapy: Theory, Research & Practice, 16*, 252–260. doi:10.1037/h0085885

Braun, V., & Clarke, V. (2006). Using thematic analysis in psychology. *Qualitative Research in Psychology, 3*, 77–101. doi:10.1191/1478088706qp063oa

Brown, D. L., Blackmon, S., & Schumacher, K. (2013). Exploring clinicians attitudes toward the incorporation of racial socialization in psychotherapy. *Journal of Black Psychology, 39*, 507–531. doi:10.1177/0095798412461806

Castonguay, L. G., Constantino, M. J., & Holtforth, M. G. (2006). The working alliance: Where are we and where should we go? *Psychotherapy: Theory, Research, Practice, Training, 43*, 271–279. doi:10.1037/0033-3204.43.3.271

Chang, D. F., & Berk, A. (2009). Making cross-racial therapy work: A phenomenological study of clients' experiences of cross-racial therapy. *Journal of Counseling Psychology, 56*, 521–536. doi:10.1037/a0016905

Connolly Gibbons, M. B., Thompson, S. M., Scott, K., Schauble, L. A., Mooney, T., Thompson, D., ... Crits-Christoph, P. (2012). Supportive expressive dynamic psychotherapy in the community mental health system: A pilot effectiveness trial for the treatment of depression. *Psychotherapy, 49*, 303–316.

Cordaro, M., Tubman, J. G., Wagner, E. F., & Morris, S. L. (2012). Treatment process predictors of program completion or dropout among minority adolescents enrolled in a brief motivational substance abuse intervention. *Journal of Child & Adolescent Substance Abuse, 21*, 51–68. doi:10.1080/1067828X.2012.636697

Cruz, M., Scott, J., Houck, P., Reynolds, C., Frank, E., & Shear, M. K. (2007). Clinical presentation and treatment outcome of African Americans with complicated grief. *Psychiatric Services, 58*, 700–702. doi:10.1176/appi.ps.58.5.700

Dattilio, F. M., Edwards, D. J., & Fishman, D. B. (2010). Case studies within a mixed methods paradigm: Toward a resolution of the alienation between researcher and practitioner in psychotherapy research. *Psychotherapy: Theory, Research, Practice, Training, 47*, 427–441.

de Roten, Y., Fischer, M., Drapeau, M., Beretta, V., Kramer, U., Favre, N., & Despland, J. N. (2004). Is one assessment enough? Patterns of helping alliance development and outcome. *Clinical Psychology & Psychotherapy, 11*, 324–331. doi:10.1002/cpp.420

Earl, T. R., Alegría, M., Mendieta, F., & Linhart, Y. D. (2011). 'Just be straight with me:' An exploration of Black patient experiences in initial mental health encounters. *American Journal of Orthopsychiatry, 81*, 519–525. doi:10.1111/j.1939-0025.2011.01123.x

Elliott, R. (2002). Hermeneutic single-case efficacy design. *Psychotherapy Research, 12*, 1–21.

Eubanks-Carter, C., Muran, J. C., & Safran, J. D. (2010). Alliance ruptures and resolution. In J. Muran & J. Barber (Eds.), *The therapeutic alliance: An evidence-based guide to practice* (pp. 74–94). New York, NY: Guilford Press.

First, M. B., Spitzer, R. L., Gibbon, M., & Williams, J. B. (1995). *Structured clinical interview for DSM-IV Axis I Disorders (SCID)*. New York, NY: Biometrics Research.

Freud, S. (1920). *A general introduction to psychoanalysis*. Oxford: Horace Liveright.

Gaztambide, D. J. (2012). Addressing cultural impasses with rupture resolution strategies: A proposal and recommendations. *Professional Psychology: Research and Practice, 43*, 183–189. doi:10.1037/a0026911

Greenson, R. R. (1965). The working alliance and the transference neuroses. *Psychoanalysis Quarterly, 34*, 155–181.

Hall, G. C. N. (2001). Psychotherapy research with ethnic minorities: Empirical, ethical, and conceptual issues. *Journal of Consulting and Clinical Psychology, 69*, 502–510. doi:10.1037/0022-006X.69.3.502

Hamilton, M. (1960). A rating scale for depression. *Journal of Neurology, Neurosurgery, and Psychiatry, 23*, 56–62. doi:10.1136/jnnp.23.1.56

Hill, C. E., Carter, J. A., & O'Farrell, M. K. (1983). A case study of the process and outcome of time-limited counseling. *Journal of Counseling Psychology, 30*, 3–18.

Horowitz, L. M., Rosenberg, S. E., Baer, B. A., Ureño, G., & Villaseñor, V. S. (1988). Inventory of interpersonal problems: Psychometric properties and clinical applications. *Journal of Consulting and Clinical Psychology, 56*, 885–892. doi:10.1037/0022-006X.56.6.885

Horvath, A. O., Del Re, A. C., Flückiger, C., & Symonds, D. (2011). Alliance in individual psychotherapy. *Psychotherapy, 48*, 9–16. doi:10.1037/a0022186

Horvath, A. O., & Greenberg, L. S. (1989). Development and validation of the Working Alliance Inventory. *Journal of Counseling Psychology, 36*, 223–233. doi:10.1037/0022-0167.36.2.223

Imel, Z. E., Baldwin, S., Atkins, D. C., Owen, J., Baardseth, T., & Wampold, B. E. (2011). Racial/ethnic disparities in therapist effectiveness: A conceptualization and initial study of cultural competence. *Journal of Counseling Psychology, 58*, 290–298. doi:10.1037/a0023284

Karlsson, R. (2005). Ethnic matching between therapist and patient in psychotherapy: An overview of findings, together with methodological and conceptual issues. *Cultural Diversity and Ethnic Minority Psychology, 11*, 113–129. doi:10.1037/1099-9809.11.2.113

Knight, Z. G. (2013). Black client, white therapist: Working with race in psychoanalytic psychotherapy in South Africa. *The International Journal of Psychoanalysis, 94*, 17–31.

Lambert, M. J., Smart, D. W., Campbell, M. P., Hawkins, E. J., Harmon, C., & Slade, K. L. (2006). Psychotherapy outcome, as measured by the OQ-45, in African American, Asian/Pacific Islander, Latino/a, and Native American clients compared with matched Caucasian clients. *Journal of College Student Psychotherapy, 20*, 17–29. doi:10.1300/J035v20n04_03

Leichsenring, F. & Schauenburg, H. (2014). Empirically supported methods of short-term psychodynamic therapy in depression–Towards an evidence-based unified protocol. *Journal of Affective Disorders, 169*, 128–143.

Luborsky, L. (1984). *The principles of psychoanalytic psychotherapy*. New York, NY: Basic Books.

Luborsky, L. (1995). Supportive-expressive dynamic psychotherapy of depression: A time-limited version. In J. P. Barber & P. Crits-Christoph (Eds.), *Dynamic therapies for psychiatric disorders* (pp. 41–83). New York, NY: Basic Books.

Luborsky, L. & Mark, D. (1991). Short-term supportive-expressive psychoanalytic psychotherapy. In P. Crits-Christoph & J. P. Barber (Eds.), *Handbook of short-term dynamic psychotherapy* (pp. 110–136). New York, NY: Basic Books.

Luborsky, L., Mark, D. Hole, A. Popp, C. Goldsmith, B., & Cacciola, J. (1995). Supportive-expressive dynamic psychotherapy of depression: A time-limited version. In J. P. Barber P. Crits-Cristoph (Eds.), *Dynamics therapies for psychiatric disorders* (pp. 13–83). New York, NY: Basic Books.

Martin, D. J., Garske, J. P., & Davis, M. K. (2000). Relation of the therapeutic alliance with outcome and other variables: A meta-analytic review. *Journal of Consulting and Clinical Psychology, 68*, 438–450. doi:10.1037/0022-006X.68.3.438

O'Farrell, M. K., Hill, C. E., & Patton, S. M. (1986). A comparison of two cases of counseling with the same counselor. *Journal of Counseling & Development, 65*, 141–145. doi:10.1002/j.1556-6676.1986.tb01261.x

Owen, J., Imel, Z., Tao, K. W., Wampold, B., Smith, A., & Rodolfa, E. (2011). Cultural ruptures in short-term therapy: Working alliance as a mediator between clients' perceptions of microaggressions and therapy outcomes. *Counselling and Psychotherapy Research, 11*, 204–212.

Owen, J., Tao, K. W., Drinane, J. M., Hook, J., Davis, D. E., & Kune, N. F. (2015, October 12). Client perceptions of therapists' multicultural orientation: Cultural (missed) opportunities and cultural humility. *Professional Psychology: Research and Practice, 47*, 30–38. doi:10.1037/pro0000046

Patton, M. J., Kivlighan, D. M., Jr., & Multon, K. D. (1997). The Missouri psychoanalytic counseling research project: Relation of changes in counseling process to client outcomes. *Journal of Counseling Psychology, 44*, 189–208. doi:10.1037/0022-0167.44.2.189

Pieterse, A. L., Todd, N. R., Neville, H. A., & Carter, R. T. (2012). Perceived racism and mental health among Black American adults: A meta-analytic review. *Journal of Counseling Psychology, 59*, 1–9. doi:10.1037/a0026208

Safran, J. D., & Muran, J. C. (1996). The resolution of ruptures in the therapeutic alliance. *Journal of Consulting and Clinical Psychology, 64*, 447–458. doi:10.1037/0022-006X.64.3.447

Safran, J. D., & Muran, J. C. (2006). Has the concept of the therapeutic alliance outlived its usefulness?. *Psychotherapy: Theory, Research, Practice, Training, 43*, 286–291. doi:10.1037/0033-3204.43.3.286

Safran, J. D., Muran, J. C., & Eubanks-Carter, C. (2011). Repairing alliance ruptures. *Psychotherapy, 48*, 80–87. doi:10.1037/a0022140

Shrout, P. E., & Fleiss, J. L. (1979). Intraclass correlations: Uses in assessing rater reliability. *Psychological Bulletin, 86*, 420–428. doi:10.1037/0033-2909.86.2.420

Stiles, W. B., & Goldsmith, J. Z. (2010). The alliance over time. In J. Muran & J. Barber (Eds.), *The therapeutic alliance: An evidence-based guide to practice* (pp. 44–62). New York, NY: Guilford Press.

Sue, D. W., Capodilupo, C. M., Torino, G. C., Bucceri, J. M., Holder, A., Nadal, K. L., & Esquilin, M. (2007). Racial microaggressions in everyday life: Implications for clinical practice. *American Psychologist, 62*, 271–286. doi:10.1037/0003-066X.62.4.271

Tao, K. W., Owen, J., Pace, B. T., & Imel, Z. E. (2015). A meta-analysis of multicultural competencies and psychotherapy process and outcome. *Journal of Counseling Psychology, 62*, 337–350. doi:10.1037/cou0000086

Vasquez, M. J. (2007). Cultural difference and the therapeutic alliance: An evidence-based analysis. *American Psychologist, 62*, 878–885.

Walling, S. M., Suvak, M. K., Howard, J. M., Taft, C. T., & Murphy, C. M. (2012). Race/ethnicity as a predictor of change in working alliance during cognitive behavioral therapy for intimate partner violence perpetrators. *Psychotherapy, 49*, 180–189. doi:10.1037/a0025751

Webster, H. B., & Bishaw, A. (2007). *Income, earnings, and poverty data from the 2006 American Community Survey*. Suitland, MD: US Department of Commerce, Economics and Statistics Administration, US Census Bureau.

Wintersteen, M. B., Mensinger, J. L., & Diamond, G. S. (2005). Do gender and racial differences between patient and therapist affect therapeutic alliance and treatment retention in adolescents? *Professional Psychology: Research and Practice, 36*, 400–408. doi:10.1037/0735-7028.36.4.400

Zetzel, E. R. (1956). Current concepts of transference. *International Journal of Psychoanalysis, 37*, 369–376.

Zilcha-Mano, S. (2017). Is the alliance really therapeutic? Revisiting this question in light of recent methodological advances. *American Psychologist, 72*, 311–325. doi:10.1037/a0040435.

The secret sorrows of men: impact of Dynamic Interpersonal Therapy on 'masculine depression'

Joanna S. Dognin and Cory K. Chen

Men are underrepresented among depression diagnoses, yet are more likely to engage in self-harm. Masculinities research has sought to better understand the mechanisms through which men may conceal or suppress depression, and has suggested that traditional diagnostic criteria may fail to recognize the many ways that gender may influence the presentation of negative affect. Ideals of hegemonic masculinity dominate military culture, making mental health treatment in a veterans' hospital an ideal setting to work through the influence of rigid gender norms on interpersonal relationships. Relational therapy can be particularly useful to help some men reconstruct their sense of self in relation to their own rigid gender norms. Dynamic interpersonal therapy is a powerful therapeutic modality that can help men recognize and connect with parts of themselves that have been previously disowned. By giving voice to these more vulnerable affects, men may be freed up to connect to and communicate their own longing for care in relationships. We will present three case vignettes to illustrate this approach among American male veterans seeking psychotherapy at a Veterans Administration (VA) Hospital in New York City.

> Every man has his secret sorrows which the world knows not; and often times we call a man cold when he is only sad. (Longfellow, 1839)

Depression in men is often hidden: while women are diagnosed with depression twice as often as men (Martin, Neighbors, & Griffith, 2013), men account for three quarters of the Western world's suicides (Seidler, Dawes, Rice, Oliffe, & Dhillon, 2016). The secret sorrows of men, as described above by the American poet Henry Wadsworth Longfellow, illustrate how – for men, sadness may be deeply buried, emotions cut-off, and depressive symptoms misunderstood as callous or cold. Connell, in her 1995 hallmark work 'Masculinities' described the impact of tightly constrained gendered norms on the emotional lives of men; her description of 'hegemonic masculinity' (Connell, 1995/2005) has influenced the field of gender studies for more than 20 years (Nascimento & Connell, 2017).

More recently, psychology literature has explored the myriad ways in which hegemonic masculine ideals may potentially complicate the identification and treatment of depression (Emslie, Ridge, Ziebland, & Hunt, 2006; Martin et al., 2013; Oliffe, Ogrodniczuk, Bottorff, Johnson, & Hoyak, 2012; Oliffe & Phillips, 2008). Hegemonic masculinity (Connell, 1995/2005) delineates rigid dichotomies between male and female, reason and feeling, and strong and weak as mechanisms to gain and maintain power (Donaldson, 1993; Roper, 1991). The experience of depression can be particularly problematic for men who resonate with such masculine ideals. In fact, the internal experience and external presentation of depression is often in direct contradiction with such ideals: tearfulness connotes femininity, powerlessness is at odds with achieving and providing, and weakness and vulnerability challenge masculine notions of self-reliance (Emslie et al., 2006). It is therefore no surprise that men experiencing depression may conceal, mask, or otherwise suppress these painful affective states.

Interpersonal approaches can be particularly useful in helping men reconstruct a valued sense of self, and to either redefine their roles within hegemonic masculinity or distance themselves from it altogether (Emslie et al., 2006). One such approach is dynamic interpersonal therapy (DIT), a time-limited (16 sessions) psychodynamic model based on a compilation of evidence-based short-term psychoanalytic/psychodynamic treatments for depression (Lemma, Target, & Fonagy, 2010, 2011a, 2011b). DIT treatment has been successfully integrated into primary care and mental health settings in the United Kingdom, Italy, Belgium, Denmark, and Holland and anticipated dissemination in China (A. Lemma, personal communication, 2016) as well as among military veterans in the United States (Chen, Ingenito, Kehn, Nehrig, & Abraham, 2017). DIT has been particularly useful in treating veterans whose rigidly defined masculine ideals interfered with their ability to form or maintain meaningful connections (Chen & Dognin, 2017).

A primary tenet of DIT is that depression, at its core, is a relational disorder. Depression occurs in response to interpersonal difficulties and perceived or real attachment threats, which lead to a threat to the self. When under threat of loss or abandonment, the depressed individual may misperceive both his own internal world and the external world around him. In the first phase of treatment, the DIT therapist works collaboratively with the patient to identify a dominant interpersonal-affective focus (IPAF), that is to say, a dominant model of relating to the self and others, which serves to reinforce the depressive symptoms. Throughout the middle phase of treatment, the patient works through his IPAF by recognizing its activation in both current significant relationships and in the therapeutic relationship, and identifying how internal affective states connect to the IPAF. The final stage of therapy allows the patient to explore and more fully understand their now-conscious affective states, and connect them to the IPAF, especially in context of the upcoming loss of the therapeutic relationship. In this phase, the DIT therapist presents the patient with a 'goodbye letter' which summarizes work completed together, describes the IPAF in relation to both challenges and successes of treatment and helps anticipate future interpersonal difficulties (Lemma et al., 2011a).

Military culture is steeped in the very notions of hegemonic masculinity and thus, ideas of what a man *should* be, feel and act dominates the themes of many

IPAFs of veterans served within our setting. Within this narrow domain, many men have had little prior experience or encouragement to reflect upon their own frame of mind. Hegemonic masculinity leaves little room for reflection and vulnerability; it lives in transactions – one controls or is controlled, one provides or is in need of provision. Yet DIT sidesteps these deeply embedded elements of *what* he thinks and feels about himself and others, and focuses instead on *how* he thinks about himself and others. The patient learns to identify how his internal models have come to influence his responses to others, and how his understandable attempts to regain stability may be fueled by misunderstandings of himself and others (Lemma et al., 2011a). In focusing on the IPAF, a patient learns to reflect on the recurring role he plays in his interpersonal narrative and collaboratively work with his therapist to shift away from a pattern of relating characterized by transactions between objects and toward an understanding of self and other as interactive subjects. The 'good-bye letter' itself may be particularly meaningful for men who have historically masked their vulnerabilities. In addition to summarizing the IPAF and course of treatment, it concretely memorializes their experiences in therapy in a way that can act as a bulwark against the urge to deny or devalue the work accomplished. The letter can function as a testament to the new experiences achieved and can help the veteran return to that place psychologically when needed. This paper further describes the relationship between depression and masculinity, and explores the clinical usefulness of DIT in facilitating greater mentalization and fostering deeper interpersonal connections among depressed male veterans seeking care in a Veterans Affairs (VA) medical center in New York City.

Depression, suicidal behavior, and masculinities

Current research in masculinities seeks to understand the gender disparity between depression diagnoses and suicide rates, and better elucidate the relationships between gender norms, and help-seeking behavior. Suicide remains a worldwide public health problem, with nearly 800,000 people completing suicide a year and scores of others making attempts. Suicide remains the second leading cause of death globally among young people (15–29) (WHO, 2018) and men are vastly overrepresented among suicide completers (Seidler et al., 2016). Among veterans in the United States (US), suicide prevention is a top priority. US veterans are 22% more likely to kill themselves than civilians; a recent report revealed that 20 veterans kill themselves a day, with the highest risk group falling on middle-to-older male adults (VHA, 2017). Understanding the inner turmoil involved in suicidal actions is difficult among men who hold these experiences so privately, and is especially crucial for therapists who may be in positions to observe or witness atypical presentations of distress.

Masculinities research has attempted to understand what emotional experiences drive suicidal behavior and what challenges exist in seeking or accepting help. One possible explanation is that hegemonic ideals discourage a man from reaching out or accepting help. Help-seeking behavior may be perceived as antithetical to being 'macho,' which may also help explain men's shorter lifespan: as they are equally unlikely to seek help for physical symptoms they take risks which may result in missing potentially dangerous medical and mental health symptoms (Oliffe & Phillips, 2008). While this explanation leaves little space for therapeutic intervention, other possible explanations may provide insight for therapists who in their practices encounter men masking their depression. First, diagnostic criteria for depression may artificially favor women by privileging symptoms they are more likely to report, such as sadness or crying (Martin et al., 2013). Second, men may acutely experience their depression differently than women. Addis proposed four conceptual frameworks which may help untangle how gender norms impact men's expression of depression: (1) *a sex differences framework*, which posits that depression is fundamentally the same illness in both women and men, and if there are differences, they are due to differences in depression rates between males and females; (2) *a masked depression framework*, that proposes that men may find expressions of weakness so unacceptable that they instead express some sort of 'depressive equivalent'; (3) *a masculine depression framework* which assumes that hegemonic masculinity encourages men to externalize their behavior and engage instead in anger, aggression, substance use, or risk-taking; or (4) *a gendered response framework*, that posits a man's expression of negative affect is influenced by how strongly he accepts or rejects hegemonic ideals (Addis, 2008). A gendered response framework suggests room for therapeutic intervention – by becoming more open to alternate views of masculinity, men in distress may have greater opportunity to identify negative affect and link this to their internal models.

In order to facilitate this, therapists may wish to consider alternative symptoms potentially present in men masking their depression. For example, Martin and colleagues developed two new scales to discern whether alternate symptom clusters exist that may help detect depression in men. The Male Symptom Scale (MSS) and the Gender Inclusive Depression Scale (GIDS) combined externalizing symptoms (aggression, substance use, and risk-taking behavior) with more traditional depressive symptoms. Conducted on data from the National Comorbidity Survey Replication, a nationally representative sample, their new scales revealed relatively equal rates of depression between males and females. Of interest, a sizable number of women also endorsed male-type depressive symptoms. While more research is needed to better distinguish symptoms of so-called masculine depression, these findings point to the need for a broader view of how sex and gender norms may influence presentation of depression (Martin et al., 2013).

Multiple masculinities, shifting gender norms, and the value of DIT

Shifting away from rigid gender norms and hegemonic masculine ideals may potentially aid in recovery from depression, and DIT is well positioned to facilitate this process. Emslie and colleagues (2006) conducted a series of qualitative interviews with men who self-identified as depressed in the United Kingdom, and found that their recovery ultimately required reconstructing a sense of self in relation to their own masculinity. Men reported that their need to feel *in control* rather than dependent impaired their ability to seek and accept help: some participants specifically cited concerns about becoming dependent on therapists or on medications for health and wellness. Hegemonic beliefs were particularly toxic, as evidenced by some participants describing suicide as an act of bravery, and incomplete suicide attempts as evidence of failure/weakness. Finally, some men in this study actively sought to distance themselves from hegemonic ideals, especially when these ideals were in direct contrast to other valued aspects of self, such as sexual orientation or racial/ethnic identity (Emslie et al., 2006). DIT may serve to allow men to examine their unconscious repeating patterns that help keep these rigid gender norms entrenched and encourage their deeper reflection on their own state of mind. In so doing, men may have the potential to loosen up some of these gender norms and experiment with new ways of being in relationship. The short-term framework of DIT may also be useful for men fearing a dependency on therapy: a collaborative, transparent, exploratory model with a clear expiration date can provide these men with the understanding and connection they crave without fears of loss of control to a therapist.

While the male participants in the above study self-identified as depressed, other men never acknowledge such feelings to others and enter clinical care only after suicidal ideation or attempts. Cleary (2012) conducted a qualitative study among 52 young males (18–30) admitted to three Dublin hospitals shortly after serious suicide attempts. In these interviews, men revealed both the extraordinary length of time they suffered internally with suicidal thoughts (generally a year or longer) as well as a reluctance to disclose these emotions to anyone within their social network. In addition to endorsing pronounced feelings of sadness and anxiety, many of the men were simply unable to label their own affective states. Those most unfamiliar with affective language tended to label their distress as physical. Most men in this study actively concealed their distress from social networks. Men reported feeling silenced by past messages shaming tears or excessive confiding in male friends. Most actually felt fearful of male friends learning of their distress, worrying that their vulnerability and emotional pain might make another male think of them as weak or feminine. Those with the strongest adherence to hegemonic masculinity sought to 'protect' important women in their lives from the depths of their despair. Many men in the study used alcohol to numb their pain, and thoughts of suicide provided welcome relief from the weight of suppressing such painful emotions (Cleary, 2012).

It is particularly notable that while men in the above study painted rich narratives of their emotional suffering, their beliefs about how men should or should not express vulnerability impeded their ability to ask for help. Yet their willingness to share their story when queried also speaks to the power of a narrative approach and potential hope for interpersonal therapy. Among a military population, Green and colleagues (2010) specifically explored how hegemonic masculinity is embedded into a soldier's identity and how this identity may impact expressions of distress. They noted an important paradox that may shed light on how dynamic therapists could help a patient reshape rigid gender norms in therapy: while becoming a solider involves adapting to hegemonic ideals of toughness and denial of vulnerability, a culture of caring and camaraderie also exists within one's team – a paradox they referred to as 'caring masculinity' (Green, Emslie, O'Neill, Hunt, & Walker, 2010). Despite clear hegemonic ideals, 'caring masculinity' was deeply embedded within military culture and provided emotional buffering in times of high stress. Therapists may be able to help draw on these stronger interdependent relationships to assist men in creating and maintaining richer and deeper relationships.

These exploratory studies in masculinities research demonstrate that gender norms are indeed malleable. While beliefs about gender roles and norms may be deeply entrenched in cultural contexts, they are subject to change. Multiple types of masculinities exist depending on one's sociocultural background, and experiences with privilege (or the lack of it). Connell's (1995) schema of masculinities incorporates hegemonic, complicit, subordinate, and marginalized forms, thus creating a foundation for intersectionality that gives us a view into how men uniquely relate to their gender identity (Connell, 1995/2005). Additionally, presentations of masculinity shift over the course of a man's lifespan, based on social and developmental expectations. For example, young adulthood is a time one focuses on establishing intimate relationships and avoiding isolation (Erikson, 1994 (reissue)). Displays of hegemonic ideals at this life stage often result in aggression, risk-taking behaviors and as a result, suicide rates and accidental deaths are particularly high. Since open displays of weakness may be discouraged among peers, many young men suppress painful emotions, isolate, and avoid seeking help when distressed (Evans, Francis, Oliffe, & Gregory, 2010).

Gender and masculinity norms intersect with race and this intersection occurs not just on an individual level but also on a systemic one. For example, Black men are a particularly vulnerable group in the US. While the mortality gap between Black and White women has closed, it has only widened between Black and White men living in America (Griffith, Metzl, & Gunter, 2011). Ideals of race, identity, and masculinity are almost entirely normed on the experience of the White man, further alienating the Black man as 'other/not belonging' before he ever sets foot in DIT treatment. For Black men, the 'provider role,' so central to hegemonic masculinity, is greatly undermined by structural racism: when compared to their White, middle-class male peers, college-educated Black men are four times more likely to experience unemployment, acquire less wealth, and be less able to move into desirable neighborhoods. For White men, educational attainment decreases the risk of suicide, yet, the opposite is true for Black men, whose suicide risk increases as they attain more education and status (Griffith et al., 2011).

Thus, gender norms can and do change, sometimes naturally over the course of one's lifespan, and other times in direct response to privileging other prominent identities such as race or sexual orientation. Gender norms also shift when one enters a new social group with set rules and mores, such as the military. As Chimamanda Ngozi Adichie, a feminist writer, argued 'culture does not make people. People make culture' (Adichie, 2017). Therefore, it is reasonable to imagine that interpersonal therapy can also loosen overly rigid and unhelpful gender norms. We will present three case vignettes[1] describing how hegemonic masculine ideals influenced DIT treatment at different points in the lifecycle, and detailing ways in which DIT can be useful in softening deeply held gender beliefs and allowing more vulnerability and connection to develop in relationships. All three cases are based on treatments that occurred in a VA medical center treating military veterans in New York City.

A portrait of the solider as a young man: intimacy vs. isolation

'Robert' is a 26-year-old, Black male referred to DIT following successful completion of Prolonged Exposure for Posttraumatic Stress Disorder (PTSD) symptoms.[2] As his PTSD symptoms resolved, Robert became more aware of an underlying depression, related to his struggles to form and maintain intimate and meaningful relationships. Following his military service, he enrolled at a prestigious university and at the time of treatment was pursuing a degree in philosophy. Robert arrived at his first session dressed in a tailored sports coat, stylish t-shirt, and jeans. He was smart, articulate, precise, and polished in his speech and thinking. He described growing up in a lower income neighborhood where his intellectual interests in philosophy, art, and chess were mocked. He felt out of place and pressured to take on a hyper-masculine and aggressive persona that did not feel genuine to him. He was shy and quiet and many of his peers found his interests unusual. As an adolescent, he was often bullied and accused of being gay. Robert identified as heterosexual but found these attacks distressing and 'emasculating.' Robert was raised by a single mother who he described as 'strong willed, intense, and demanding.' A prominent memory of his consisted of an instance when he was accused of starting a fight with another boy at school. Robert remembered with pride his mother standing up to a white schoolteacher, defending his honesty. While Robert respected his mother, he also found her intimidating and sometimes frightening. Robert recalled his mother's rage toward him when he stole a candy bar from a convenience store at age 5. Although this went unseen by the store clerk, his mother struck him repeatedly with a belt when she discovered his misdeed.

Over the course of the therapy, Robert began to recognize his mother's fear for her son. His mother made very clear to Robert the unforgiving dangers of being a Black man in America. From these experiences with his mother, Robert developed a fear of expressing aggression, particularly in contexts where that aggression may be perceived as threatening (e.g. when interacting with law enforcement where an officer's perception of aggression could endanger his life). Growing up, he witnessed a friend beaten by the police in a case of mistaken identity. No action was taken following the officers 'mistake.' Robert described feeling both frightened and enraged at the ease with which government agents could act on those in his community with impunity, but he felt forced to hide this rage, particularly in his current school setting. He described frequently feeling out of place in this context as well, noting that he had been repeatedly stopped and questioned by campus police regarding his status as a student at his university. Robert had no difficulty meeting women – Robert recognized that he was often initially perceived as attractive, intelligent, and polished; however, he described these encounters as short-lived relationships which inevitably ended when the women became frustrated by his 'aloofness' and 'passivity.' Over time, Robert was able to recognize that he often viewed himself as an unappreciated outsider to a judgmental and threatening other. Robert attempted to navigate his relationships by hiding himself and wearing a polished mask of indifference but Robert himself frequently felt anxious and depressed about the repeated rejections he suffered. Over the course of therapy, Robert was able to recognize that his passivity served multiple functions – an overgeneralized strategy originally designed to demonstrate his 'harmlessness' in the context of a society with limited tolerance for his aggression; a demonstration of fidelity to the lessons his mother taught him; and a way to manage the intense rage he experienced about the racism he experienced. Robert was eventually able to recognize that this strategy blunted his emotional experience in ways that left him disconnected from himself and others. Treatment worked to reconnect Robert with his feelings, validate the sources of his anger, and find ways of giving voice to his anger, particularly in relationships where the lack of connection to his feelings resulted in alienation from others (Figure 1).

Overt displays of hegemonic masculinity are complicated for men of color, and Robert's case demonstrates the intersection between race and oppression, depression, and masculinities. As a Black male growing up in a poor neighborhood, he has received a plethora of messages to dial down his natural sensitivity and intelligence (feminine traits) and amp up his more aggressive ones (masculine traits). Yet this message is fraught with conflict, as depicted by his early experiences with his mother. As tough as his neighborhood is, he is painfully aware that his masculinity is marginalized and outright displays of anger or aggression are viewed through a racial lens of the 'angry Black male,' further increasing his risk of harm. Not accepted for his truer intellectual/sensitive side and faced with conflicting messages, Robert adapts a cool (not too hot or cold) front, which requires him to suppress rage, sadness, and vulnerability. Consequently, he views his self to be an 'unappreciated outsider' to a cruel and judgmental other, and his very aloofness both protect him and elicit the same rejection he fears. Through DIT treatment, he was able to reconnect with and accept a fuller range of emotions, which allowed him to experiment with being more connected in relationships.

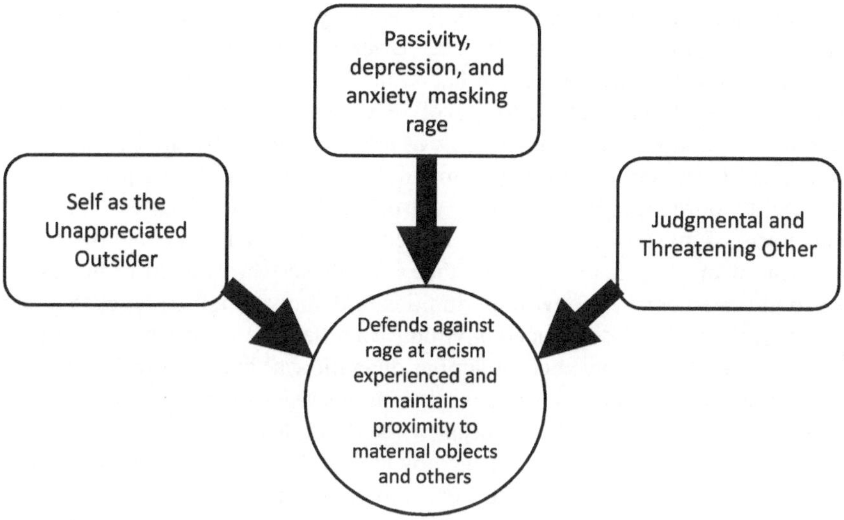

Figure 1. IPAF for Robert.

Middlemarch: generativity vs. stagnation

'Brian' is a 47-year-old, White male who was referred by his Primary Care doctor for depression and interpersonal conflict. During the first session, Brian launched into a litany of complaints about the burden of needing to 'save the day' for the various irresponsible and incompetent people in his life. Brian's mother had been chronically depressed and unable to function for months at a time. Brian's father was often away, struggled with alcoholism, and was only sporadically employed. From an early age, as the oldest of three children, Brian ensured his siblings were cared for and fed. The lack of employment opportunities in his community led Brian to enlist in the Army (although he later acknowledged it as an effort to escape his family circumstances). While in the Army, Brian reveled in the experience of having his needs attended to by the military. He advanced quickly and enjoyed the sense of reciprocity as he took care of those under his command. However, after his military service, Brian often found himself frustrated with civilians who he considered 'incompetent, uninformed, and undisciplined.' He often found himself 'taking over' at the first signs that the other person was not performing to his standards, a pattern that caused significant conflict in his professional and personal life.

Through DIT, Brian came to recognize that he viewed himself as the 'responsible caretaker' who was burdened with compensating for 'irresponsible/ incompetent others.' When others did not meet his expectations, Brian would 'take charge' to solve the problem. While part of him enjoyed his status as 'the savior' and felt needed and valued, Brian also grew more aware of his motivation to avoid potential disappointment. 'I don't want to give anyone the opportunity to fail me in the way that my parents did.' Brian became tearful in session as he recalled his seventh birthday. Brian had waited with gleeful anticipation for his parents to present him with the toy revolver and sheriff's badge he had hinted at wanting for months. Brian's horror grew as the hours ticked by and he realized his parents had forgotten his birthday completely. 'What kind of parent just forgets their child's birthday?' Brian recalled, 'From that day on, I learned I just need to take care of myself.' The therapist helped Brian to see that he had become so proficient at meeting his own needs that even those who wanted to be responsive to him were left with few opportunities to demonstrate their care. 'My wife often complains that I don't need anything from her and it makes her feel like I could just take her or leave her.' A similar dynamic was explored within the therapy relationship. Brian often brought material to sessions having already 'figured out what was going on' with a solution worked out, leaving the therapist feeling uninvolved and unnecessary. Brian acknowledged that his strategies for avoiding vulnerability and dependency also kept him from getting the attentiveness and care for which he longed. Brian eventually disclosed his fears that his only value to the people in his life was as a caretaker. As Brian was better able to access and articulate his feeling of disappointment, sadness, and longing in the therapy room, he was encouraged to share these feelings with his wife and begin experimenting with being more than the 'caretaker' in their relationship. In the final sessions of the therapy, Brian described his wish to continue treatment and his sadness at its end. The therapist helped Brian to recognize that his ability to acknowledge and express this desire was itself a significant achievement and communicating these desires had the potential to make his other relationships rewarding and meaningful in ways he had rarely experienced (Figure 2).

Being a productive member of society is the main developmental task of adulthood's middle phase. It is a time of focus on career/work, of developing more responsibility, and of providing for one's family and loved ones. Middle adulthood is also a time when emotional energy is focused on providing stability and producing something of value (Erikson, 1994 (reissue)). Rigid adherence to male gender roles may exacerbate these desires to provide, especially in someone conditioned to be the 'caretaker,' who may lack the capacity to accept such caring for him. Since masculine identity is so focused on the 'provider role,' the work a man does, his status and income may become inextricably wrapped up in his self-worth. Rigid adherence to hegemonic masculinity often results in men at this stage ignoring their body's cues to slow down, leading to increased injury or disability, which then triggers feelings of vulnerability and threats to this prized provider identity. For men whose jobs require hard physical labor, denial of physical strain or pain may lead to greater injury. Similarly, for men in white-collar industries, hegemonic ideals may favor the 'hardy man' – the man in control; yet this very focus on achievement and being in control may lead one to ignore physical signs of stress and become more vulnerable to coronary events. It is therefore

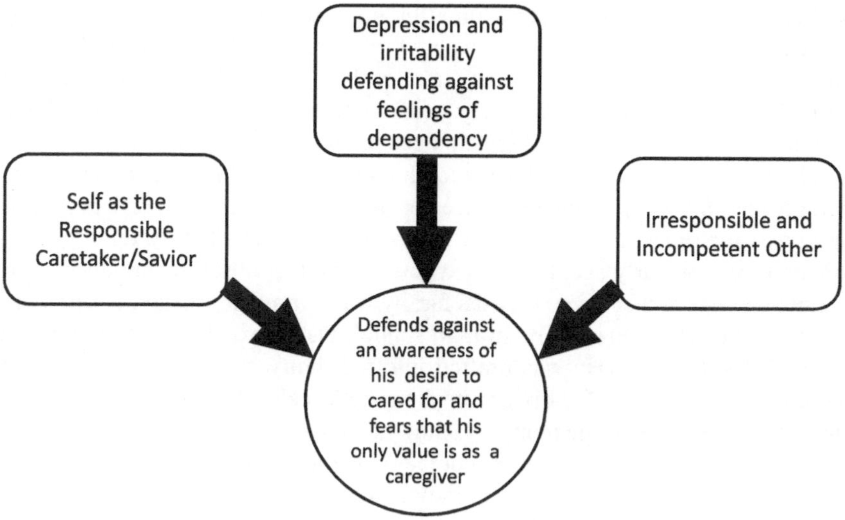

Figure 2. IPAF for Brian.

of little surprise that depression rates and veteran completed suicides peak at this life stage, and that correlations between hegemonic masculinity and depression are especially pronounced in middle age (Evans et al., 2010).

Emotionally, something even more insidious may be intensifying Brian's need to provide. Brian's early childhood experiences with a depressed mother and an alcoholic, absent father left his emotional needs neglected. Adapting in childhood to a very hegemonic masculine ideal of caretaker provided him early status as the male provider who is always in control. The military served a protective function by exchanging achieving for real caring among a band of brothers (an example of the 'caring masculinities' discussed earlier). Yet outside the structured military environment, Brian struggled to develop a sense of mutual caring in his relationships and continued to replay the sad and empty role of a hyper-competent provider to an incompetent/irresponsible other. By walling off his vulnerable self from the pain of disappointment, he inadvertently was contributing to this dynamic by not letting anyone see or attempt to meet his needs, thus denying any possibilities of true mutuality. Through therapy, Brian was better able to connect to the sad and vulnerable self who longed for care and experiment with new ways to elicit such caring.

Lives of quiet desperation: integrity vs. despair

'David' is a 78-year-old, recently widowed, Hispanic male, referred by the geriatric clinic for interpersonal difficulties with family and VA staff. David's adult children were exasperated by his unwillingness to follow the medical team's advice regarding diet, physical activity, and medications. On measures of depression and anxiety, David denied every item on both scales, but the medical team that had worked with David for many years, noticed a more withdrawn and subdued demeanor and suspected these changes related to the recent loss of his wife. David's refusal to abide by medical recommendations for chronic but manageable health conditions was putting him at greater risk for other serious health problems. David was the oldest child in a large extended family. His family ran a grocery store and from an early age, he was expected to help at the store and oversee his younger siblings and cousins. David's family was warm and loving but often harried from struggling financially. In high school, David excelled in sports, which he recalled with pride. He was drafted into the Army during the Vietnam War where he was respected for his physical strength, calm demeanor, and thoughtfulness in taking care of the men he commanded. After discharge from the Army, David started his own construction company. He met and married his wife soon after returning from the military and they had three children. David and his wife had remained healthy for much of their lives together and he continued to work into his early 70s. David grinned with pride as he remembered the surprise of those who worked for him when he would occasionally help at construction sites – swinging a sledgehammer as a 70-year-old. However, when David was 75, his wife was diagnosed with cancer. David retired to focus on caring for his wife, who died three years later.

Initially, David described his relationships cheerfully – proud of the role he played in the military, at work, and in his own family. He saw himself as 'calm and in control,' frequently managing the crises of others or allaying their fears. David chuckled at the memory of his wife becoming 'hysterical' when their 5-year-old daughter had disappeared during a family picnic. David recalled soothing his wife and calmly thinking through where his daughter might be. He soon found her at a carousel just a few yards away. David now characterized his adult children and the medical team's concerns as 'hysterical.' The therapist and veteran reflected on the ways being 'calm and in control' was reinforced across many contexts of his life. David also acknowledged that he often viewed others as 'hysterical' and unnecessarily anxious. Over time, David began to recognize other feelings that arose at the times he was 'calm and in control.' He associated to a memory of himself as a 10-year-old boy, supervising his two younger siblings and a 1-year-old cousin. His cousin had started crying and David had no idea how to comfort her. In an effort to not scare his younger brother and sister, David had forced himself to appear calm and in control but he now recalled feeling terrified. David came to acknowledge that his bravado was a mask he wore to calm others. He tearfully described his struggle to retain this mask as he reassured his wife after her diagnosis and hid his feelings of terror and powerlessness.

As David's capacity to tolerate and give voice to these vulnerable aspects of his experience increased, he became more aware of the sadness, loss, and vulner-

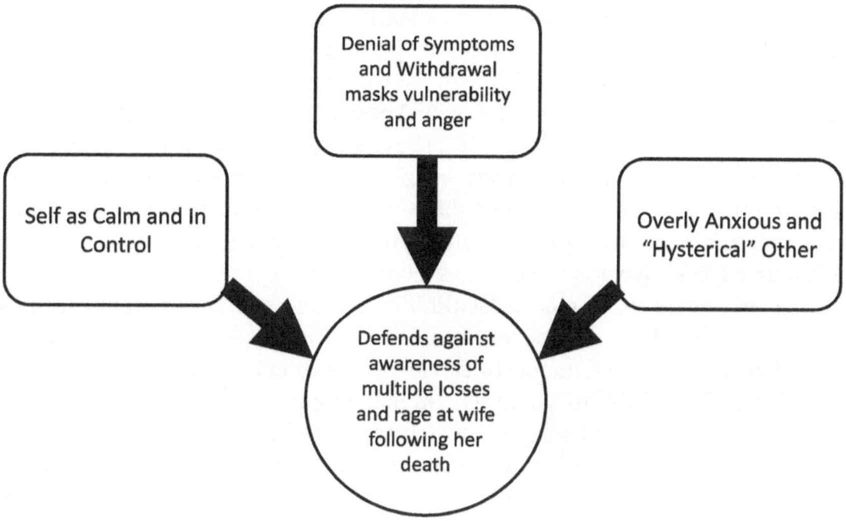

Figure 3. IPAF for David.

ability he felt following the death of his wife. He also guiltily admitted feeling resentful toward his wife at being forced to retire from his work, resulting in a loss of his sense of self-worth and identity. David became more aware of the physical changes he was experiencing and his desire to deny them. He admitted avoiding physical activities because it made him acutely aware of what he was no longer able to do and just how much weaker he had become. David's therapist helped him to recognize that by presenting himself as unperturbed, the other people in his life were forced to 'hold' all of the anxiety, which perpetuated his view of them as 'hysterical.' David came to recognize the ways this was playing out with his family and medical team. As David began to acknowledge his anxiety and depression, the scores on these measures increased; however, David felt that these scores represented a more realistic and honest reflection of his inner experience. The increased acknowledgment of his distress also paralleled David's increased capacity and willingness to accept the medical care he needed. Finally, in his relationship with his children and grandchildren (who had been hurt and confused by his aloofness at their mother's death), David began to acknowledge and mourn the significant losses in his life and in doing so, was able to connect more deeply and genuinely than he ever had before (Figure 3).

Older adulthood is a particularly vulnerable time for many men and maintaining hegemonic ideals becomes a great deal harder at this life stage. The conflict between integrity and despair (Erikson, 1994 (reissue)) is most prominent, with despair resulting in substantially higher acts of completed suicides compared to older women (Conwell, Van Orden, & Caine, 2011). Many factors conspire together to threaten one's sense of masculinity: the physical body declines and becomes frayed, and career/work loses its prominence, leading to a sense of loss of control, connections, and visibility in the world (Evans et al., 2010). In a qualitative analysis of 77 depressed older men, Apesoa-Varano and colleagues referred to this as the 'shamed masculine self.' They posited that older men experienced shamed masculinity related to their inability to perform their usual manhood tasks, and that their defense against this shame was to either behave even more overtly masculine or to further isolate themselves from social interactions that elicit shame (Apesoa-Varano, Barker, & Hinton, 2015).

Themes related to shamed masculinities underscored David's clinical presentation as well. His wife's death, loss of work-related identity and status and physical decline all posed threats to David's sense of masculinity and contributed to his depression. Since his youth, David had adopted a mask of being cool and collected – 'the strong silent type,' which was reinforced in the military, in his family and at work. His alignment with hegemonic masculinity was characterized by stoicism and disconnection from his affect. As the benefits reaped by this stance began to disintegrate, David began withdrawing from social interaction. Therapy helped David increase his awareness into the costs of this retreat and helped him reconnect to the vulnerability underneath his aloofness, which stemmed from terror over the loss of control and the unknown. While gaining access to this vulnerability increased his conscious experience of depression and anxiety, this access also allowed him to mourn the loss of his wife and previous life and redefine his sense of self in relation to his masculinity.

Conclusion

Depression in men often goes underreported, a potentially dangerous situation given increased risk of interpersonal isolation and suicide. Adherence to rigid gender norms may so profoundly distance men from their internal suffering that they may be disconnected from their own affect. Others deeply experience internal turmoil but suffer it in silence, stifled by the weight of ideals about how men should or should not express their distress. These patterns have devastating impacts on relationships throughout the life cycle and are particularly amenable to interpersonal therapy. A DIT framework has the capacity to help men connect with, validate, and give voice to feelings that are usually disowned. By being more connected to these feelings, they are better able to connect more deeply with those in their interpersonal life. As therapy helps to loosen these rigid gender norms, men are freed up to connect with their longing and need to be cared for, and ask for – and allow, others to care for them. By acknowledging their vulnerability, they can be more open to seeking needed medical and mental health care.

Disclosure statement

No potential conflict of interest was reported by the authors.

Funding

This work was supported by American Psychoanalytical Association and International Psychoanalytic Association to train psychologists in Dynamic Interpersonal Therapy (DIT).

Notes

1. Cases presented are an amalgamation of several patient cases. All identifying information has been changed to protect identity of patients in treatment.
2. Prolonged Exposure (PE) for Posttraumatic Stress Disorder is an evidenced-based treatment for PTSD that is used throughout Veterans Affairs hospitals in the US.

References

Addis, M. E. (2008). Gender and depression in men. *Clinical Psychology: Science and Practice, 15*, 153–168.

Adichie, C. (2017). *We should all be feminists*. New York, NY: Alfred A. Knopf.

Apesoa-Varano, E. C., Barker, J. C., & Hinton, L. (2015). Shards of sorrow: Older men's accounts of their depression experience. *Social Science & Medicine, 124*, 1–8. doi:10.1016/j.socscimed.2014.10.054. Retrieved from https://www.ncbi.nlm.nih.gov/pubmed/25461856

Chen, C. K., & Dognin, J. S. (2017). Addressing the influence of hegemonic masculinity on veterans through brief dynamic interpersonal therapy. *Psychology of Men & Masculinity, 18*(3), 238–242. doi:10.1037/men0000118

Chen, C. K., Ingenito, C. P., Kehn, M. M., Nehrig, N., & Abraham, K. S. (2017). Implementing brief Dynamic Interpersonal Therapy (DIT) in a VA Medical Center. *Journal of Mental Health*, 1–8. doi:10.1080/09638237.2017.1340602. Retrieved from https://www.ncbi.nlm.nih.gov/pubmed/28699818

Cleary, A. (2012). Suicidal action, emotional expression, and the performance of masculinities. *Social Science & Medicine, 74*(4), 498–505. doi:10.1016/j.socscimed.2011.08.002. Retrieved from https://www.ncbi.nlm.nih.gov/pubmed/21930333

Connell, R. (1995/2005). *Masculinities* (2nd ed.). Berkeley: University of California Press.

Conwell, Y., Van Orden, K., & Caine, E. D. (2011). Suicide in older adults. *Psychiatric Clinics of North America, 34*(2), 451–468, ix. doi:10.1016/j.psc.2011.02.002. Retrieved from https://www.ncbi.nlm.nih.gov/pubmed/21536168

Donaldson, M. (1993). What is hegemonic masculinity? *Theory and Science, 22*, 643–657.

Emslie, C., Ridge, D., Ziebland, S., & Hunt, K. (2006). Men's accounts of depression: Reconstructing or resisting hegemonic masculinity? *Social Science & Medicine, 62*(9), 2246–2257. doi:10.1016/j.socscimed.2005.10.017. Retrieved from https://www.ncbi.nlm.nih.gov/pubmed/16289741

Erikson, E. H. (1994 (reissue)). *Identity and the life cycle*. New York: W.W. Norton & Company.

Evans, J. B., Francis, B., Oliffe, J. L., & Gregory, D. (2010). Health, Illness, Men and Masculinities (HIMM): A theoretical framework for understanding men and their health. *Journal of Men's Health, 8*(1), 7–15.

Green, G., Emslie, C., O'Neill, D., Hunt, K., & Walker, S. (2010). Exploring the ambiguities of masculinity in accounts of emotional distress in the military among young ex-servicemen. *Social Science & Medicine, 71*(8), 1480–1488. doi:10.1016/j.socscimed.2010.07.015. Retrieved from https://www.ncbi.nlm.nih.gov/pubmed/20739109

Griffith, D. M., Metzl, J. M., & Gunter, K. (2011). Considering intersections of race and gender in interventions that address US men's health disparities. *Public Health, 125*(7), 417–423. doi:10.1016/j.puhe.2011.04.014. Retrieved from https://www.ncbi.nlm.nih.gov/pubmed/21724208

Lemma, A., Target, M., & Fonagy, P. (2010). The development of a brief psychodynamic protocol for depression: Dynamic Interpersonal Therapy (DIT). *Psychoanalytic Psychotherapy, 24*(4), 329–346. doi:10.1080/02668734.2010.513547

Lemma, A., Target, M., & Fonagy, P. (2011a). *Brief dynamic interpersonal therapy. A clinician's guide*. New York, NY: Oxford University Press.

Lemma, A., Target, M., & Fonagy, P. (2011b). The development of a brief psychodynamic intervention (dynamic interpersonal therapy) and its application to depression: A pilot study. *Psychiatry, 74*(1), 41–48. doi:10.1521/psyc.2011.74.1.41. Retrieved from https://www.ncbi.nlm.nih.gov/pubmed/21463169

Longfellow, H. W. (1839). *Hyperion*. Boston, MA: Samuel Colman.

Martin, L. A., Neighbors, H. W., & Griffith, D. M. (2013). The experience of symptoms of depression in men vs women: Analysis of the National Comorbidity Survey Replication. *JAMA Psychiatry, 70*(10), 1100–1106. doi:10.1001/jamapsychiatry.2013.1985. Retrieved from https://www.ncbi.nlm.nih.gov/pubmed/23986338

Nascimento, M., & Connell, R. (2017). Reflecting on twenty years of Masculinities: An interview with Raewyn Connell. *Ciência & Saúde Coletiva, 22*(12), 3975–3980. doi:10.1590/1413-812320172212.27242016. Retrieved from https://www.ncbi.nlm.nih.gov/pubmed/29267714

Oliffe, J. L., Ogrodniczuk, J. S., Bottorff, J. L., Johnson, J. L., & Hoyak, K. (2012). 'You feel like you can't live anymore': Suicide from the perspectives of Canadian men who experience depression. *Social Science & Medicine, 74*(4), 506–514. doi:10.1016/j.socscimed.2010.03.057. Retrieved from https://www.ncbi.nlm.nih.gov/pubmed/20541308

Oliffe, J. L., & Phillips, M. J. (2008). Men, depression and masculinities: A review and recommendations. *Journal of Men's Health, 5*(3), 194–202. doi:10.1016/j.jomh.2008.03.016

Roper, M. T. J. (1991). *Manful assertions*. London: Routledge.

Seidler, Z. E., Dawes, A. J., Rice, S. M., Oliffe, J. L., & Dhillon, H. M. (2016). The role of masculinity in men's help-seeking for depression: A systematic review. *Clinical Psychology Review, 49*, 106–118. doi:10.1016/j.cpr.2016.09.002. Retrieved from https://www.ncbi.nlm.nih.gov/pubmed/27664823

VHA. (2017). *VA releases veteran suicide statistics by state*. Retrieved from https://www.va.gov/opa/pressrel/includes/viewPDF.cfm?id=2951

WHO. (2018). *Suicide*. Retrieved from http://www.who.int/mediacentre/factsheets/fs398/en/

‘Post-natal’ depression in fathers, or Early Fatherhood Depression

Sameer P. Sarkar

Both men and women are known to suffer from post-natal depression. However, there has been little attention paid to the psychodynamic genesis of post-natal depression in fathers. In this paper, I describe case histories of post-natal depression in two first time fathers and offer a formulation for understanding post-natal depression in such cases. I suggest a range of reasons for the failure to recognize this condition; and possible therapeutic interventions.

Introduction

A vast literature exists on the nature of motherhood, both in academic and popular discourse. Films, books and TV programmes address the experience of motherhood in comedy, drama, science, and historical genres. By contrast, fathers are often treated as largely absent or jokey figures, with many sit-coms contrasting a smart, active mother with a foolish and incompetent father figure. Children’s films show a similar pattern; mothers and stepmothers are present in Disney films from their beginning in 1934, but no fathers appear as main characters in a movie until the Lion King in 1994. Similarly, Pixar’s massively successful ‘Toy Story’ series depicts a family with no father and no mention of one; it is not until ‘Finding Nemo’ in 2003 that the father character has a pivotal and positive role. While in real life an expectant mother often gets a polite and affectionate inquiry on her visible ‘baby bump’, such as if it is her ‘first time’ or if the sex of the unborn is known yet, fathers can claim no such attention. In the ‘mother-infant’ dyad, there is no place for the father who is seen as the ultimate outsider.

Ross (1979) wrote that ‘until recently the father has been the forgotten parent in psychoanalytic and psychological literature’. Treatment of fathers in psychoanalytic literature has been limited to the ‘absent father’, ‘the father as the Oedipal myth’ and ‘the father whom the mother made’. Happily however, fatherhood and fathering have recently become interesting again for psychoanalysts after decades of preoccupation with mothers and mothering (Trowell & Etchegoyen, 2002).

In this paper, I will focus on the psychological experience of fatherhood, and review the literature available. I specifically discuss the psychological risk factors for post-natal depression in fathers and describe via brief clinical materials (case summaries) where paternal post-natal depression was the clinical focus. I suggest possible reasons why paternal post-natal depression might be ignored or overlooked; and suggest implications for treatment. Although the condition is being increasingly recognized, the fact that we still lack proper terminology even to describe the phenomenon (e.g. male postpartum depression or early fatherhood depression) somewhat supports the contention about the clinical neglect of this condition.

A caveat though to start with. Paternal post-natal depression, much like maternal post-natal depression, is not phenomenologically much different from any other variety of depression. The array of symptoms is essentially the same, the treatment similar and the outcome not dissimilar. Save the time when post-natal mood disorder evolves to the more serious 'post-partum psychosis', which incidentally has also been reported in fathers (Shapiro & Nass, 1986), there is little to distinguish the so called PND (post-natal depression) from non-childbirth related depression. Besides the unique temporal relationship with the ordinary physiological act of giving birth (or adoption in rare cases), it may be worth examining if the classification of post-natal depression as a separate clinical entity has any nosological significance, or any validity. The same, however, can be said of much of the current diagnostic classification system in psychiatry as a whole although it is generally accepted that diagnostic labels carry the useful function of being a form of 'medical shorthand'.

The general point above about the lack of validity of psychiatric diagnoses is not meant to suggest that we should not give sufficient weight to the specificity of maternal PND, which develops not only in response to processes of pregnancy and lactation, but also in connection with the complex unconscious fantasies which accompany these processes. With regard to the latter however, I would argue in this paper that fathers are not immune to the complex unconscious fantasies and its role in the genesis of depression in post-natal period.

Background: post-natal depression

Post-natal psychiatric distress and morbidity (in both parents) is recognized in a wide variety of cultures and countries, although not all societies recognize it as a medical disorder (Oates et al., 2004). The commonest form of post-natal disorder is post-natal depression which is recognized to occur in both men and women (Ballard & Davies, 1996; Paulson & Bazemore, 2010). The prevalence of post-natal depression in women in the first six months after giving birth is about 25%, whereas for men, the figure is about 10%. The incidence of significant depression among new fathers has been estimated to be between 1.2 and 25.5% (Paulson & Bazemore, 2010).

Risk factors for post-natal depression in men include depression in their partner, a difficult and unloving relationship with their partner and a previous history of depression (Bielawska-Batorowicz & Kossakowska-Petrycka, 2006; Goodman, 2004). These risk factors resemble the risk factors for women, where lack of social support and a confiding relationship and a previous history of depression are known to be risk factors for post-natal depression (Stein, Cooper, Campbell, Day, & Altham, 1989). Post-natal depression in men may develop during their partner's pregnancy; and is associated with changes to the family structure and loss of sexual intimacy (Condon, Boyce, & Corkindale, 2004). Paulson (2010) believes there is growing evidence suggests that paternal depressive symptoms are predicted by interpersonal problems with the mother and maternal depressive symptoms.

The most severe form of depressive disorder that occurs after birth is post-natal affective psychosis, which occurs in 1:500 deliveries. Although post-natal psychosis is thought to be initiated by rapid changes in maternal hormone levels in the immediate post-partum period, cases of post-partum psychosis have been reported in men (Shapiro & Nass, 1986). Suicide and filicide are rare behaviors associated with post-natal psychotic disorders. Quevedo et al. (2011) assessed 650 men for suicide risk in the antenatal period and within 30–60 days post-partum. They found the prevalence of suicide risk in this period for fathers was 4.8%.

The effects of post-natal depression in fathers can be damaging not only for the men themselves but for their families, and the optimal development of their children's mental health. Lamb (2010) first described the importance of the father in the child's development, describing the equal attachment of children to both mothers and fathers from 6 months of age. Grossmann, Grossmann, Fremmer-Bombik, Kindler, and Scheuerer-Englisch (2002) and Grossmann, Grossmann, Kindler, and Zimmermann (2008) report the importance of the father's ability to play with their children in children's development. It is therefore not surprising that a longitudinal study of child development that measured paternal post-natal depression found that it was associated with behavioral disturbances in children, especially oppositional defiant disorder in sons (Ramchandani, O'Connor, et al. (2008; Ramchandani, Stein, et al., 2008).

Cultural accounts of fatherhood

Like motherhood, fatherhood is as much a social construct as it is a psychological experience. Becoming a father therefore entails an engagement with social constructions of gender role and masculinity, as well as role change with the social and family networks. Just as for mothers, the experience of becoming a father is likely to be profoundly influenced by an individual's social, cultural, and ethnic norms, as well as his own experience of being parented (Matthey, Barnett, Ungerer, & Waters, 2000).

In many cultures and across historical traditions, masculinity and fatherhood are entwined concepts. Fatherhood has been associated with protection of the home and family culture, as opposed to hands-on care of children or the home, which is seen as women's work (Ferree, Lorber, & Hess, 1999; Roopnarine et al.,

1995). Fatherhood is also sometimes associated with the delivery of discipline, which may be accompanied by threat or punishment. Many traditional societies are called 'patriarchal' in recognition of the fact that they are dominated by fathers who 'own' the families they are responsible for; which includes 'ownership of both wives and their off-spring' (Wilson & Daly, 1995).

Cultural expectations of fathers changed in late twentieth century Western cultures, perhaps in response to changes in feminine gender role expectations, and the status of women in twentieth century western society. Within some classes and ethnic groups, fathers caring for the children is no longer thought of as a violation of masculine sex role norms, nor an indication of abnormal feminine characteristics in a male. In these cultures, accordingly, the cultural definition of masculinity is also changing (Blum, 2004; Branney & White, 2008; Franklin II, 2012).

For any parent, a baby may represent pride and accomplishment, a restatement of the parent's gender identity and confirmation of their sex role; and an opportunity to improve upon the past, and provide this baby with an upbringing that is as good as the parent had, or better. But if a new parent's conscious memories of childhood are complicated and painful, then a new baby maybe seen as a rival, a sibling, a reminder of past trauma, a new burden or a loss of opportunity or role (Blum, 2007; Knowles, 1990; Knowles & Cole, 1990).

Just as for mothers, the role of 'father' may mean different things to different people; not all of them positive. Ross (1995; cited in Blum, 2004) describes a range of possible paternal responses:

- Uncertainty about his identity as a father and the actual role of a father
- A changed relationship to his wife
- A changed relationship with his family of origin
- Revival of oedipal rivalries and conflicts
- Revival of pre-oedipal, symbiotic (and oral) longings
- Sudden arousal of maternal and feminine identifications and anxieties about these identifications
- A sense of personal limits and injury along with the contrary possibility of self-extension and immortality through one's legacy
- A new internal relationship to one's own father
- The need to integrate object representations of the child and self- representation in the role of the father

These experiences may not occur in all men; and they may be transitional and resolvable for most. It seems likely that those men who experience the most negative appraisals of a child and the role of father are more likely to be those men whose own fathers reacted negatively to them, and/or who had relationships with their own fathers characterized by fear or distress.

Psychoanalytic views about fathers

Early psychoanalysts did view the father as the central figure in mental life. Freud described the 'oedipal' dilemma for a male child as a competition between the boy and his father for the mother's attention. Others, like Ferenczi and Abraham, focused on the major role of the 'castration complex' as a major organizer for emotional growth. Their theoretical outlook, in keeping with the times, were patrocentric and phallocentric. In the classical Oedipal situation, the son experiences the father as rival or threat, and this is not resolved until the son gives up his attachment to the mother, and turns his emotional gaze outside the family. Most boys manage this successfully but a persistent competition with father for women's attention is likely to lead to neurotic distress.

Freud wrote little about the experience of fatherhood; although it is of interest that fathers feature commonly in his case histories (Little Hans, The Rat Man) (Freud, 1955), and he himself had a close paternal relationship with his daughter Anna. His uncritical view of traditional and conventional theories of masculinity and its social roles has been the subject of some criticism by later feminist psychoanalysts (Connell & Connell, 2005) and social scientists (Smiler, 2004). Freud's theoretical position was that maternal and paternal function is largely instinctual; although he was one of the first to argue that all humans have bisexual elements to their personality. However, he made no distinction between sexual identity, gender identity, gender role expectations, and erotic object choices, all of which are thought to be environmentally influenced (Butler, 2011; Connell, 1989; Lorber & Farrell, 1991; Stoltenberg, 1990).

Later writers have suggested that Freud omitted to consider that the father may be jealous of the attention paid by the mother to the child (Jordan & Wall, 1993; Tammentie, Paavilainen, Åstedt-Kurki, & Tarkka, 2004). Evidence from animal studies of non-human primates suggests that although some aspect of maternal and paternal behavior is innate, much parental care-giving is determined by an interaction of genetic profile with environmental experience (Harlow, 1958; Suomi, 1995). In many animal species, fathers are an active threat to their offspring, especially if they block access to females. Human fathers may have to learn to manage feelings of hostility toward their children that arise out of jealousy (Reeb, Conger, & Wu, 2010). A major collaborative work compiled by Trowell and Etchegoyen (2002), almost a hundred years after Freud expressed his seminal views on the role of fathers, remains the most definitive reference volume on the psychoanalytic re-evaluation of importance of fathers. Presented as a gift by a thoughtful colleague on the day my first child was born, this book first inspired me to attempt to write this essay.

The psychodynamics of parenting: relevance of attachment

After World War II, the rapid evolution of psychoanalytic knowledge, including object relations theories, ethnology, and direct observational studies on child development, resulted in an increase in interest in the mother-child dyad and the study of motherhood as a developmental phase. Melanie Klein and Anna Freud in UK, and Margaret Mahler in the US, wrote about the infant's dependence on the mother and conflicts over separation and individuation. In the 1960s, studies of attachment relationships in humans have provided empirical evidence for Freud's claim that early childhood relationships with parents affect the development of adult attachment relationships with peers and partners (Bowlby, 1960). Animal studies have found that early attachments to peers and parents influence the development of the neocortex, affect, and arousal systems (Kraemer, 1992; Schore, 2000, 2002a, 2002b). In humans, the development of cognitive representations of attachment relationships not only influences affect and arousal regulation, but also the development of cognitive models of the self, and self-reflective function (Fonagy, Steele, Steele, Moran, and Higgitt 1991; Schore, 2000, 2001, 2002a, 2002b).

Babies develop attachments to fathers as well as mothers (Lamb, 1977, 2010) and form internal working models of both parents (Grossmann et al., 2008). It is known that mothers' attachment representations predict their children's attachment patterns with 75% accuracy (Fonagy et al., 1991). Fathers' attachment patterns also influence their children's attachment behavior (Grossmann et al., 2008).

Studies of attachment in mothers have found that adult maternal attachment representations influence maternal behavior toward their child. Mothers with insecure attachment representations may struggle to care for their offspring (Lyons-Ruth, Bronfman, & Parsons, 1999; Schuengel, Bakermans-Kranenburg, & Van IJzendoorn, 1999) an effect that may be mediated through the release of affiliative neuropeptides, such as oxytocin (Strathearn, Iyengar, Fonagy, & Kim, 2012). If maternal attachment representations affect a woman's experience of becoming a mother and providing maternal care, then it is plausible that a man's attachment representations may influence his experience of becoming a father and providing paternal care.

It may be that the attachment representation acts as a cognitive appraisal system through which events are experienced and judged as threatening or stressful. Individuals with insecure attachment models are more likely to appraise the world as frightening or stressful (McMahon, Barnett, Kowalenko, & Tennant, 2005) Insecure adult attachment representations are associated with adult psychopathology and are over-represented in clinical populations (Bakermans-Kranenburg & van IJzendoorn, 2009).

The influence of adult attachment representations has been studied in relation to the development of post-natal depression in women; and so may be relevant to paternal post-natal depression. The well-known Camberwell studies of Brown and Harris (1978) found women who had histories of ruptured attachments to their mothers had an increased risk of depression, especially if they had a demanding maternal role, and a lack of a confiding relationship. Women who develop post-natal depression are more likely to have fearful attachment patterns than women who do not develop post-natal depression or PND (Bifulco et al., 2004; McMahon et al., 2005).

Psychodynamic formulations of post-natal depression in men: a tentative model

There has been considerable discussion of women's transition to motherhood from a psychoanalytic perspective. Significant writers on this subject include Winnicott (1948), Deutsch (1945), Stern (2009), Pines (1978) and Raphael-Leff (1991). Besser, Vliegen, Luyten, and Blatt (2008) summarize and review the psychoanalytic literature on post-natal depression; emphasizing the work of Blatt (1974) who argues that post-natal depression is a likely consequence when there is an unresolved tension between autonomy and dependency.

Blum (2007) describes three key emotional areas of conflict that may give rise to post-natal depression: dependency and the mother's own need for care; her anger with the baby and related guilt; and conflicts with her identity as a mother, based on her experience of being cared for by her own parents. Both Blatt and Blum's work are mirrored by the research into a new mother's representation of her own attachment experiences with her mother; and how this impacts on her relationship with the baby (Grossmann et al., 2008).

However, to date there do not appear to be any psychodynamic accounts of post-natal depression in men. The clinical examples given below are intended not as evidence of the model offered (which, if possible at all, would require much more extensive presentation of clinical material) but an illustration of it. I attempt to describe the model with reference to Blum (2007) and Besser et al. (2008) and their discussions of PND.

The cases of Mr. Benjamin Button and Jason Bourne[1]

Over the years, I have seen in treatment scores of otherwise previously healthy military personnel from the three services (and Royal Marines) in the British Armed Forces (and for a period, the US Air Force) as well as civilians who presented with developing depressive symptoms following childbirth. The degree of severity ranged from what would be otherwise equivalent to 'post-partum blues' in mothers, to severe depression with psychotic features. Although described in literature, I have not seen a single case among fathers that could be considered to be equivalent to 'post-partum psychosis' in mothers. In my own clinical practice I have found the prevalence of post-natal depression in either parents to be roughly the same. From this large and varied cohort I picked the two cases, (one each from civilian and military background) below for their uniqueness of circumstances, severity of symptoms and relatively long period in treatment.

Mr. Button

Mr. and Mrs. Button are a highly successful, professional, married couple, both aged 40 years. The decision to have a child was mutually agreed but not carefully thought out. The pregnancy and child-birth were largely uneventful save for the anxiety and uncertainties faced by both after conception while genetic tests to detect congenital abnormalities were underway. Due to their advanced age, the fetus was considered to be 'high risk' in terms of genetic and developmental disorder associated with increased maternal age at conception. Mrs. Button did not experience any mood symptoms during pregnancy or in the post-natal period. Both were medically healthy and free of psychological symptoms prior to the birth of the child. Shortly after birth, Mrs. Button went abroad with the infant on maternity leave to her own parents. Mr. Button accompanied them on the trip but returned home after two weeks.

Due to their work commitments in different cities far apart, and the need to reside near their workplaces, Mr. Button, with great deal of ambivalence, took on the hands-on care of the baby just when the baby was weaned off mother's milk. Mr. Button, unfamiliar as he was with the care of a new born, managed to juggle a heavy work-load of a high-stress, high-responsibility senior position with child-care, amply supported by local friends and a crèche at work. Mrs. Button would visit over the weekends. Neither had any extended family locally to speak of.

As the infant grew, Mr. Button became depressed with prominent somatic symptoms and frequent death wishes. At the peak of his depression he actively considered driving his car off a cliff, or into oncoming traffic (without the child) but always resisted at the thought of the implications it would have on the child. He could not tolerate the thought of leaving the child with no carer for any extended period of time before his disappearance was discovered. In his words: 'I could not imagine the child waking up, crying, and no one to come to him. Imagine what would that be for a helpless infant'.

Mr. Button did seek help, initially with a counselor, and then took antidepressants with reduction of suicidal thoughts. He made some unwise choices in his personal relationships which led to trouble at work and eventual dismissal. His dismissal was eventually overturned by High Court. All through his struggles, his wife remained unaware of his mental condition or difficulties at work. He self-referred to therapy through a program that assists professionals in crisis.

Mr. Button's own infancy somewhat mirrors that of his child. His own father was absent when he was born, having emigrated to a neighboring country for a better life, ostensibly for his family. As an infant, he was raised by his very young mother in a large extended family where child care was shared among many women. In a rural agrarian society, the males in the household where Mr. Button was raised for the first 18 months of his life confined themselves to the occasional horse-play with the baby. It is suspected that his mother was depressed although it was not detected or treated as such.

When he was a child about 20 months old, Mr. Button's mother, spurred on by the fact that his father had made no attempt to see him or send for them, illegally crossed the border under cover of night with just the infant and no belongings and appeared where she knew her husband was residing. The reunion surprised his father but they quickly settled in their new family life. At age 8, the Button child was sent to an expensive all-male boarding school where he would finish his schooling before undertaking further professional and higher studies. He would say that he 'never really knew my siblings' although he had three other siblings, none of whom went to boarding school.

Mrs. Button came from a family of highly successful professionals and is from the same ethnic and national background as her husband. She was very close to her two sisters who were also close in age to her. Raised mainly by nannies and governesses, the sisters formed a deep close personal bond which limited their exposure to any meaningful peer group until much later in adulthood. Prior to marrying Mr. Button, she did not have any significant relationships.

In therapy, Mr. Button often talked about: 'I was not born to wash and sterilize milk bottles (referring to milk bottles for the infant)'. He said his main motivation to seek help was 'not wanting to spend a fortune in therapist fees for the child when he is all grown up'. Once rid of suicidal ideas/death wishes, he frequently talked about 'superman complex' (I can do anything and do it well) and 'caring for a baby is not rocket science- women do it' but alternated this feeling of 'greatness' with deep self-loathing. His hostility toward his wife in particular and women in general was barely concealed. His relationship with his siblings was strained and although he was a dutiful son, the eldest in the family, his relationship with both his parents was deeply conflicted with equal measure of guilt for 'not being there' and resentment for being leaned on by his entire family for support.

Mr. Bourne

Mr. Bourne, a military officer in his early 30s and married to a civilian banker 4 years his junior, presented with symptoms of depression (including somatic symptoms) that appeared after the birth of their first child. Both were of previously good health and came from a background of relative affluence, him of generations of distinguished military service and the only child, her of finance and banking, and also an only child. The child was planned, even carefully timed to take advantage of relaxing and rather generous parental leave entitlements.

Mr. Bourne expressed a degree of pride in being of the 'generation' when gender equality was thought to be not only desirable, but achievable and wanted to 'play his part'. As a 'hands-on dad', he participated with equal vigor in the care of the infant although admitted in treatment sessions that he feared that he was not doing a 'good enough' job. He did cop a fair degree of criticism from his family and close friends for his involvement in the day to day aspect of child care. He talked, with a degree of irony, about one of his close friend jokingly suggesting that he should somehow establish that the baby is 'allergic to latex' (reference to the material of the teat or 'nipple' of the feeding bottle) so that he can be 'out of the loop' when it came to preparing feed for the infant at night time.

He complained about lack of sleep (and consequent tiredness all next day) although his wife took more responsibility for the infant during the nights, since he did go back to work after the 10 days' paternity leave. He reported changes in the relationship with his wife after the birth which became increasingly poor. He often thought about divorce and said that they stayed together only for the infants' sake. In sessions he described more conflicts, arguments, irritations, and frustrations between him and his wife than before and the relationship became strained, small things became big, they misunderstood each other, and many problems remained unsolved. He felt that they did not communicate with each other as they had done before and when they communicated they often talked through the infant. At the same time, his relationship with his own parents deteriorated after he felt that his mother, a rather strict and 'regimented military wife' was taking the side of his wife and devaluing his 'sacrifices' while his father continued to disparage him for getting involved in practical child care duties as 'new age nonsense'. He experienced that love disappeared and he often referred to the impairment of the relationship with his wife as an explanation of his depressed mood.

As he started to experience symptoms of low mood which first appeared a week after the birth deteriorating, he tried to fight them by increasingly getting involved with the daily care of the infant. Determined to make 'shared-parenting' work, he met the conflicting priorities in his life by developing rigid routines, constantly negotiating with his wife, and reprioritizing to try find time of his own, albeit unsuccessfully. He saw this reverting to routines as a strategy to get balance back into life, and felt that hope for the future was to wait for better times. This passivity, inability to prioritize, and to deal with the situation as it presented itself might have been an outcome of his depressive symptoms. As his depression deepened, his care of the child became chaotic to the point of being essentially excluded from any child care duties by his parents and wife. Relieved, he went back to work and his symptoms gradually resolved.

Discussion

Mr. Button's case neatly explicates the themes described by Blatt (1974) and Blum (2007). He described the demands of looking after a small baby; demands that he had never had to deal with before, and which involved close physical and emotional contact with a small boy. He was giving care at home and had a responsible job during the day: but there was no-one to care for him. His baby son was entirely dependent on him; a responsibility which he both valued and feared. He struggled with intense ambivalence feelings of hostility and love toward a small version of himself. His relationship with his wife was ambivalent and complex and he did not feel supported by her; at the same time he felt guilty about resenting her. He struggled with dependency needs, anger and an abrupt transition to the role of fatherhood that neither his childhood experience nor his cultural background had prepared him for. His attachment to therapy was also ambivalent, and he experienced his first therapists as trying to con or demean him.

Mr. Bourne on the other hand revealed a healthier attachment history compared to Mr. Button and he arguably suffered less symptoms. He never was suicidal and much of his resentments were centered on the 'mixed messages' society was sending him which included the denigration by his father and the unforgiveable alignment of his mother, whose approval he sought, with his wife. While his father's derision of him was understandable from the generational viewpoint, his mother's 'betrayal' was seen as abandonment which made him regress to a helpless infant. The feeling that his own child was anything but 'abandoned' receiving the best attention from both parents only heightened his sense of injustice.

Dependency

Men who experience profound and persistent ambivalence toward their children may become depressed as they alternate between feeling love and tenderness toward their child, oscillating with hostility, hatred, anger, and frustration. This may be hard enough if there are no other new demands on the father; as Condon et al. (2004) points out, the loss of spousal intimacy is depressing for many new fathers. However, if the father also has to actually take on the physical care of the baby (because the mother is not physically available for whatever reason), then he may have to manage conflicting feelings toward his son or daughter while being physically responsible for their well-being.

The experience of negative feelings toward a loved person is distressing for anyone; but especially for those men and women who struggled with managing anger, sadness, and despair before the birth of a child. These men and women will struggle with the normal feelings of rage and distress that can accompany parenthood (Winnicott, 1964), and may experience profound guilt which manifests as depression.

Resentment of a vulnerable child can give rise to a deep depression. In Mr. Button's case, he experienced his baby's distress as 'The baby just hates me'; which then he elaborated as 'I am no good as a nurturer, so the baby hates me'. We may also speculate that Mr. Button projected his own hatred of the baby's distress, experiencing it as an attack and increasing his anxiety. Sometimes Mr. Button described experiencing his baby son as ungrateful and demanding, and verbalized this as 'He sucks the life out of me'. We see here again an identification with his own depressed (and possibly suicidal) mother; and also the experience of his son as a threat to his own life. The phrase also suggests an anxiety that the baby literally could not suck (life-sustaining milk) from him; and that he was a biologically inferior carer. Similar feelings about an inferior parent are also expressed by Mr. Bourne who felt that he always had to comply with what his wife told him to do regarding the care of the infant. Although Mr. Button was essentially a single-parent he also felt like Mr. Bourne in experiencing their partners as evaluating and criticizing them when they cared for the infant, and felt that they were not allowed to be fathers in their own way.

In patriarchal cultures, vulnerability is associated with low status and being treated with contempt; and may stimulate feelings of fear in a parent. Cultural issues may also be relevant, especially for migrant families who are not able to engage in the usual cultural practices around child care. Men who migrate from countries where there is a strongly patriarchal culture where fathers are not hands-on carers may be uncomfortable if they move into new cultures where men are expected to participate in child care. There is then the possibility of cultural cognitive dissonance amplifying and magnifying psychological distress. Cultural expectations of the masculine may exclude any acknowledgment of dependency longings, and this type of machismo does not support reflection on early childhood attachment experience and neediness. Some fathers may see their sons getting a type of care and attention that they never had, and experience acute envy and rage (Bergman & Hobson, 2002). Both the fathers in the examples above, despite their vastly different backgrounds and personal circumstances, perceived that society gave them contradictory messages about equality in parenthood, since mothers always were seen as the head parent. Both expressed their frustration that the role of the father is poorly defined and since the traditional role as a breadwinner no longer exists, fathers today serve as proxy, whose role is exchangeable, and thus, fathers are not seen as important as mothers.

Where dependency needs have not been met in childhood, an adult may sublimate their needs for care by becoming a carer, for example, a health care professional (Bowlby, 1960). However, this counter-dependent adaptation may not work well for those who have unresolved dependency issues where dependency is seen as a weakness and must be disavowed. This may be a particular issue for single parents, who are faced with the task of doing all the caring for themselves as well as a baby. Any normally competent individual who can ordinarily juggle all life demands of them may break down when faced with the feelings of 'there is no one to take care of me', but there may be a particular problem for those individuals with unresolved dependency issues who find themselves having to be single parents. They are more vulnerable and need more help than those who are more ready to acknowledge their own dependency needs, but tragically may be least able to ask.

A man with unresolved dependency needs may find fatherhood especially anxiety provoking and distressing. This anxiety and distress may be compounded if he lacks a spousal companion to support him; and if he has increased responsibilities in relation to baby care. Men who cannot tolerate closeness may find that a baby invites closeness like no other person; and therefore generates intense anxiety.

Ross (1979) suggested that maternal, nurturing identifications are threatening to masculine identity, but Bergman and Hobson (2002) suggest that maternal identification can support identity. A man who has a secure sense of his own masculinity will not be threatened by his own maternal capacity and femininity; whereas a man whose masculine identity feels unsafe and insecure may find the maternal role uncomfortable and anxiety provoking. The identification process is influenced by attachment models and may therefore be profoundly affected by the man's early experiences of being fathered and mothered.

Miller (2002) and Blum (2004) both note that a baby can act as a transference object who can generate fantasies and expectations in any parent (including those who are not genetically related to the child). However, the parental relationship with the baby is also one in which the past is replayed in the present, and parents play out their own experiences with their fathers and mothers. If these past experiences are largely secure ('good enough', in Winnicott's immortal phrase), then this is what the father will bring to the relationship. If he recalls himself as a 'difficult' child or if he has a difficult (and unresolved) attachment to his own mother, the investment in the child may become over-compensatory and clinging, or angry and rejecting. Either way the relationship in such cases can become so fragile that an ordinary infant's demands can then become the proverbial straw that breaks the camel's back.

Anger

The role of anger in the genesis of depression is well-known. Besser et al. (2008) and Gilbert et al. (2008) emphasize the importance of self-directed criticism and hostility in the generation of depression, including post-natal depression. A father who is angry with his baby son is more likely to be angry with himself; and at risk of internalizing his anger and feeling suicidal; as Mr. Button did. Such pathological anger may also be displaced and externalized onto other persons and although happily this did not happen to Mr. Button, in other fathers, violent attacks on partners may occur for the first time in pregnancy and in the post-natal period. Fathers who become depressed often have traditional, stereotyped gender role identities, such as that a man should be strong, successful, always in control, and capable of handling problems without help. The 'Superman complex' of Mr. Button was really a barely compensated defense against the insecurity of not being in control and doing a terrible job as a parent. Both these fathers who felt depressed postpartum, might have the 'hegemonic masculinity' as an ideal characterized by emotional control and lack of vulnerability and thus incompatible with their feelings of lack of control and powerlessness for how men should be.

Anxiety and fear about what might happen if angry feelings were expressed can lead to anger being directed inward, further lowering self-esteem, creating a vicious cycle. Brownhill, Wilhelm, Barclay, and Schmied (2005) describe 'the big build' as a description of the relationship between male depression, hostility, and violence to self or others. Men first attempt to avoid, then numb and then escape their psychological pain. When there is no escape, the pain becomes a mixture of hatred and hurt, which is finally acted out as self-harm or harm to others.

This model may have utility for understanding Mr. Button's post-natal depression. His anxiety about how to care for his child was unavoidable and inescapable. As his anxiety and distress mounted, it became a mixture of hatred and guilt at feeling so hostile toward a defenseless child. The unacceptability of anger toward the child and the guilt at expressing anger leads to self-criticism and self-loathing which then leads to a depressed position. The inwardly directed anger, not only at the child but also all those associated with the child, (for example, the child's mother) may give rise to a feeling of tremendous failure (to contain one's anger) and then to repression of the anger and guilty self-reproach. This anger, if not processed appropriately, can take the form of acting out by being unduly harsh on the child or by withdrawing from the child which then would hinder formation of a healthy attachment. Failure to manage anger toward the child may explain the increased risk of anxiety disorders in sons of depressed fathers (Ramchandani, O'Connor, et al., 2008; Ramchandani, Stein, et al., 2008).

Emasculation fantasy

Although fatherhood can be (and biologically is) masculinity affirming, there is also the fear and fantasy of being emasculated. I suggest that this is more common in men who develop depression in the post-natal period where symbolically the baby is the one who emasculates him by taking away his companions, work and hobby and turn him into a 'woman'; who like a woman (and mother) automatically assumes the caring role without thinking. In treatment both fathers often talked about having to sacrifice all their interests and social life to the priority of the child.

They said they missed leisure time, time to be together with their wives, and to see friends. They missed their work and work-mates when they were on parental duty, and their baby and family when they were working. Blum (2004) suggests that much of our stereotypic view of masculinity is a defense against early acquired femininity, and identification with mother. What happens when the overt masculinity is neutralized by the sleep disturbance caused by the odd sleep wake cycle of a baby? Or taking care of the unpredictable incontinence of its excretions? Or the regurgitation of milk which reminds him of his own helpless state?

The day a child is born is seen by some fathers as the 'first day of the rest of your life'. This idealized fantasy is played out in the identification with the man's own father, who may have been a shadow of his former self, weighed down by the demands of family and fatherhood, and being the breadwinner. For Mr. Button, his own father may have become a 'toothless tiger' on whom it was increasingly difficult to direct oedipal hatred. The guilt that followed was then linked with the vision that Mr. Button was becoming the same 'toothless tiger'; an object of pity not hatred, having been emasculated by the twin demands of new found role of nurturance and perpetuity of being the provider. Many of a man's ordinary pursuits that occupied him before his child is born are by necessity curtailed or even totally forgotten with these twin demands not only from the child but from his mother whose demands take a different form. Demands no longer only of love and affection but a demand, however muted, that the childcare is shared or even taken over by him. Although intending to be an equal parent, the fathers above felt deviant in their father role, and furthermore, they reported that others in their environment also saw them as deviant fathers.

The absence of breast which may have been a comfort (as nourishment is not possible) now becomes a source of resentment as the man realizes that for all the caring and nurturing he does, a vital link is missing. Not being physiologically possible, there is no intimate link between him and the baby in a physical connection through the breast or the womb. As the twin absence of the biological physical connection is internalized, the conflict between the emasculation in a psychic sense (becoming a woman) and the envy of breast in a physical sense grows which can give rise to unresolved anger that festers, and later may manifest as a profoundly depressed position.

Conclusion: fatherhood and motherhood

Mr. Button's case provides some clinical evidence that assumption of the maternal role may be a risk factor for post-natal depression in some men, just as it is for women. Being placed in the maternal role activates internal working models of the early relationship with one's own mother; especially how she responded to the need for soothing and care. Any experience of not feeling cared for, or of maternal lack of interest, may be incorporated into a working model of closeness to others, which, when activated, causes anxiety and agitation. The sense of abandonment shared by both Mr. Button's mother and himself possibly gave rise to the insecure attachment which manifested itself in his distorted sense of self and self-worth. A man with such insecurity of attachment who is then asked to provide care for a child may experience anxiety ('how can I give care that I did not have?') that can build into self-loathing ('I am not good enough to care about'). This ambivalent and insecure attachment can also give rise to a heightened sense of duty (and morality) which guards against the very painful possibility of abandonment of the child and the inevitable guilt that follows. By itself, on one hand this can be a hugely protective facet, yet a painful burden on the other, akin to a self-flagellating super-ego that does not soothe but only punishes.

Mr. Button may also have experienced jealousy of his wife's attention to his son and of his son's enhanced care compared to his own. Men with insecure attachment histories may become jealous of their own children, a jealousy which can be enacted as violence to their partner and hostility to the child. Even Mr. Bourne who had shared the parental duty equally felt that the mothers' opinions were seen as more important than the father's by the health care personnel and the society. It is possible that they may also have felt jealous of their son's attachment to their partners; and his anxiety that the baby preferred her care to his: as if the baby rejected him for his wife, the more successful parent.

The cases above illustrate that the chief implications for therapy are the importance of therapist awareness, and the need to explore changes in attachment systems in new male referrals. I would suggest that this is highly pertinent to work in the NHS, especially in primary care, where front-line workers such as health visitors and community midwives could promote greater awareness of depression or depressive features during early fatherhood and of their potential impact on the infant's emotional development (regardless of whether the father is the main carer).

Dependency and vulnerability in male patients are still sometimes overlooked as stereotypes of gender and sex role by the therapist as well as the patient. It is also crucial for the therapist to inquire sensitively about suicide risk as well as thoughts of violence to the mother and the baby.

Acknowledgments

I am grateful to Dr. Gwen Adshead, teacher and friend, who not only helped improve the clarity of the first draft, but also provided endless hours of discussion, and peer-supervision on parenting, so vital to our work with the Family Courts. This paper would not be possible without her unwavering support and help throughout my own journey into fatherhood. My most sincere gratitude also to the two anonymous reviewers whose astute observations, and thoughtful comments I have tried to incorporate as best as I could. Those invaluable comments have taught me much.

Disclosure statement

No potential conflict of interest was reported by the author.

ORCID

Sameer P. Sarkar http://orcid.org/0000-0002-5410-488X

Note

1. Fictitious name used to protect identity.

References

Bakermans-Kranenburg, M. J., & van IJzendoorn, M. H. (2009). The first 10,000 Adult Attachment Interviews: Distributions of adult attachment representations in clinical and non-clinical groups. *Attachment & Human Development, 11*(3), 223–263.

Ballard, C., & Davies, R. (1996). Postnatal depression in fathers. *International Review of Psychiatry, 8*(1), 65–71.

Bergman, H., & Hobson, B. (2002). Compulsory fatherhood: The coding of fatherhood in the Swedish welfare state. In B. Hobson (Ed.), *Making Men into Fathers: Men, Masculinities, and the Social Policies of Fatherhood.* New York, NY: Cambridge University Press.

Besser, A., Vliegen, N., Luyten, P., & Blatt, S. J. (2008). Systematic empirical investigation of vulnerability to postpartum depression from a psychodynamic perspective: Commentary on issues raised by Blum (2007). *Psychoanalytic Psychology, 25*(2), 392–410.

Bielawska-Batorowicz, E., & Kossakowska-Petrycka, K. (2006). Depressive mood in men after the birth of their offspring in relation to a partner's depression, social support, fathers' personality and prenatal expectations. *Journal of Reproductive and Infant Psychology, 24*(1), 21–29.

Bifulco, A., Figueiredo, B., Guedeney, N., Gorman, L. L., Hayes, S., Muzik, M., ... Henshaw, C. A. (2004). Maternal attachment style and depression associated with childbirth: Preliminary results from a European and US cross-cultural study. *British Journal of Psychiatry, 184*(S46), s31–s37.

Blatt, S. J. (1974). Levels of object representation in anaclitic and introjective depression. *The Psychoanalytic Study of the Child, 29*(1), 107–157.

Blum, L. D. (2004). The baby as a Transference object for the father: Discussions of Bergman's chapter "The Experience of Becoming and Being a New Father". In S. Akhtar & H. Parens (Eds.), *Real and imaginary fathers: Development, transference, and healing* (pp 164–184). Lanham, MD: Jason Aronson.

Blum, L. D. (2007). Psychodynamics of postpartum depression. *Psychoanalytic Psychology, 24*(1), 45–62.

Bowlby, J. (1960). Ethology and the development of object relations. *The International Journal of Psycho-analysis, 41*, 313–317.

Branney, P., & White, A. (2008). Big boys don't cry: Depression and men. *Advances in Psychiatric Treatment, 14*(04), 256–262.

Brown, G. W., & Harris, T. (1978). *Social origins of depression*. London: Tavistock.

Brownhill, S., Wilhelm, K., Barclay, L., & Schmied, V. (2005). 'Big build': Hidden depression in men. *Australian & New Zealand Journal of Psychiatry, 39*, 921–931.

Butler, J. (2011). *Gender trouble: Feminism and the subversion of identity*. New York, NY: Routledge.

Condon, J. T., Boyce, P., & Corkindale, C. J. (2004). The first-time fathers study: A prospective study of the mental health and wellbeing of men during the transition to parenthood. *Australian and New Zealand Journal of Psychiatry, 38*(1–2), 56–64.

Connell, R. W. (1989). Making gendered people: Bodies, identities, sexualities. In M. M. Ferree, J. Lorber, & B. B. Hess (Eds.), *Revisioning gender* (pp. 449–472). Thousand Oaks, CA: Sage.

Connell, R. W., & Connell, R. (2005). *Masculinities*. Berkeley: University of California Press.

Deutsch, H. (1945). *The psychology of women: A psychoanalytical interpretation* (Vol. 2). Motherhood, NY: Grune and Stratton.

Ferree, M. M., Lorber, J., & Hess, B. B. (1999). *Revisioning gender* (Vol. 5). Lanham, MD: Rowman Altamira.

Fonagy, P., Steele, M., Steele, H., Moran, G. S., & Higgitt, A. C. (1991). The capacity for understanding mental states: The reflective self in parent and child and its significance for security of attachment. *Infant Mental Health Journal, 12*(3), 201–218.

Franklin II, C. W. (2012). *The changing definition of masculinity*. New York, NY: Springer Science & Business Media.

Freud, S., Strachey, A., & Tyson, A. (1955). *Standard edition of the complete psychological works of Sigmund Freud*, volume X (1909): Two case histories ('Little Hans' and the 'Rat Man'). London: Hogarth Press.

Gilbert, P., McEwan, K., Mitra, R., Franks, L., Richter, A., & Rockliff, H. (2008). Feeling safe and content: A specific affect regulation system? Relationship to depression, anxiety, stress, and self-criticism. *The Journal of Positive Psychology, 3*(3), 182–191.

Goodman, J. H. (2004). Paternal postpartum depression, its relationship to maternal postpartum depression, and implications for family health. *Journal of Advanced Nursing, 45*(1), 26–35.

Grossmann, K., Grossmann, K. E., Fremmer-Bombik, E., Kindler, H., & Scheuerer-Englisch, H. (2002). The uniqueness of the child–father attachment relationship: Fathers' sensitive and challenging play as a pivotal variable in a 16-year longitudinal study. *Social Development, 11*(3), 301–337.

Grossmann, K., Grossmann, K. E., Kindler, H., & Zimmermann, P. (2008). A wider view of attachment and exploration: The influence of mothers and fathers on the development of psychological security from infancy to young adulthood. In J. Cassidy & P. R. Shaver (Ed.), *Handbook of attachment: Theory, research, and clinical applications* (2nd ed., pp. 857–879). New York, NY: Guilford Press

Harlow, H. F. (1958). The nature of love. *American Psychologist, 13*(12), 673.

Jordan, P. L., & Wall, V. R. (1993). Supporting the father when an infant is breastfed. *Journal of Human Lactation, 9*(1), 31–34.

Knowles, J. P. (1990). Woman-defined motherhood. *Women & Therapy, 10*(1–2), 1–7.

Knowles, J. P., & Cole, E. (1990). *Motherhood: A feminist perspective*. New York, NY: Haworth Press.

Kraemer, G. W. (1992). A psychobiological theory of attachment. *Behavioral and Brain Sciences, 15*, 493–511. doi:10.1017/S0140525X00069752

Lamb, M. E. (1977). The development of mother-infant and father-infant attachments in the second year of life. *Developmental Psychology, 13*(6), 637–648.

Lamb, M. E. (Ed.). (2010). *The role of the father in child development*. New York, NY: Wiley.

Lorber, J., & Farrell, S. A. (Eds.). (1991). *The social construction of gender* (pp. 309–321). Newbury Park, CA: Sage.

Lyons-Ruth, K., Bronfman, E., & Parsons, E. (1999). Chapter IV. Maternal frightened, frightening, or atypical behavior and disorganized infant attachment patterns. *Monographs of the Society for Research in Child Development, 64*, 67–96.

Matthey, S., Barnett, B., Ungerer, J., & Waters, B. (2000). Paternal and maternal depressed mood during the transition to parenthood. *Journal of Affective Disorders, 60*(2), 75–85.

McMahon, C., Barnett, B., Kowalenko, N., & Tennant, C. (2005). Psychological factors associated with persistent postnatal depression: Past and current relationships, defence styles and the mediating role of insecure attachment style. *Journal of Affective Disorders, 84*(1), 15–24.

Miller, L. J. (2002). Postpartum depression. *JAMA, 287*, 762–765.

Oates, M. R., Cox, J. L., Neema, S., Asten, P., Glangeaud-Freudenthal, N., Figueiredo, B., … Yoshida, K. (2004). Postnatal depression across countries and cultures: A qualitative study. *British Journal of Psychiatry, 184*(S46), s10–s16.

Paulson, J. H. (2010) *Focusing on depression in expectant and new fathers*. Retrieved April 20, 2017, from http://www.psychiatrictimes.com/major-depressive-disorder/focusing-depression-expectant-and-new-fathers

Paulson, J. F., & Bazemore, S. D. (2010). Prenatal and postpartum depression in fathers and its association with maternal depression. *JAMA, 303*(19), 1961–1969.

Pines, D. (1978). On becoming a parent. *Journal of Child Psychotherapy, 4*(4), 19–31.

Quevedo, L., da Silva, R. A., Coelho, F., Pinheiro, K. A. T., Horta, B. L., Kapczinski, F., & Pinheiro, R. T. (2011). Risk of suicide and mixed episode in men in the postpartum period. *Journal of Affective Disorders, 132*(1–2), 243–246.

Ramchandani, P. G., O'Connor, T. G., Evans, J., Heron, J., Murray, L., & Stein, A. (2008). The effects of pre-and postnatal depression in fathers: A natural experiment comparing the effects of exposure to depression on offspring. *Journal of Child Psychology and Psychiatry, 49*(10), 1069–1078.

Ramchandani, P. G., Stein, A., O'Connor, T. G., Heron, J. O. N., Murray, L., & Evans, J. (2008). Depression in men in the postnatal period and later child psychopathology: a population cohort study. *Journal of the American Academy of Child & Adolescent Psychiatry, 47*(4), 390–398.

Raphael-Leff, J. (1991). *Psychological processes of childbearing*. London: Anna Freud Centre.

Reeb, B. T., Conger, K. J., & Wu, Y. (2010). Paternal depressive symptoms and adolescent functioning: The moderating effect of gender and father hostility. *Fathering: A Journal of Theory, Research, and Practice about Men as Fathers, 8*(1), 131.

Roopnarine, J. L., Brown, J., Snell-White, P., Riegraf, N. B., Crossley, D., Hossain, Z., & Webb, W. (1995). Father involvement in child care and household work in common-law dual-earner and single-earner Jamaican families. *Journal of Applied Developmental Psychology, 16*(1), 35–52.

Ross, J. M. (1979). Fathering: A review of some psychoanalytic contributions on paternity. *Internat. J. Psycho-Anal, 60*, 317–327.

Ross, J. M. (1995). Freud and forbidden knowledge. *Journal of the American Psychoanalytic Association, 43*, 553–571.

Schore, A. N. (2000). *Foreword to the reissue of attachment and loss, vol. 1: Attachment by John Bowlby*. New York, NY: Basic Books.

Schore, A. N. (2001). The right brain as the neurobiological substratum of Freud's dynamic unconscious. In D. Scharff (Eds.), *The psychoanalytic century: Freud's legacy for the future* (pp. 61–88). New York, NY: Other Press.

Schore, A. N. (2002a). The self-organization of the right brain and the neurobiology of emotional development. In M. D. Lewis & I. Granic. *Emotion, development, and self-organization: Dynamic systems approaches to emotional development* (pp. 155–185). New York, NY: Cambridge University Press.

Schore, A. N. (2002b). Clinical implications of a psychoneurobiological model of projective identification. *Primitive Mental States, 2*, 1–65.

Schuengel, C., Bakermans-Kranenburg, M. J., & Van IJzendoorn, M. H. (1999). Frightening maternal behavior linking unresolved loss and disorganized infant attachment. *Journal of Consulting and Clinical Psychology, 67*, 54–63.

Shapiro, S., & Nass, J. (1986). Postpartum psychosis in the male. *Psychopathology, 19*(3), 138–142.

Smiler, A. P. (2004). Thirty years after the discovery of gender: Psychological concepts and measures of masculinity. *Sex Roles, 50*(1/2), 15–26.

Stein, A., Cooper, P. J., Campbell, E. A., Day, A., & Altham, P. M. (1989). Social adversity and perinatal complications: Their relation to postnatal depression. *BMJ, 298*(6680), 1073.

Stern, D. N. (2009). *The first relationship*. Cambridge, MA: Harvard University Press.

Stoltenberg, J. (1990). *Refusing to be a man: Essays on sex and justice*. New York, NY: Meridian/ Penguin.

Strathearn, L., Iyengar, U., Fonagy, P., & Kim, S. (2012). Maternal oxytocin response during mother–infant interaction: associations with adult temperament. *Hormones and Behavior, 61*(3), 429–435.

Suomi, S. J. (1995). Influence of Bowlby's attachment theory on research on nonhuman primate biobehavioral development. In S. Goldberg, R. Muir, & J. Kerr (Eds.), *Attachment theory: Social, developmental, and clinical perspectives* (pp. 185–201). Hillsdale, NJ: Analytic Press.

Tammentie, T., Paavilainen, E., Åstedt-Kurki, P., & Tarkka, M. T. (2004). Family dynamics of postnatally depressed mothers–discrepancy between expectations and reality. *Journal of Clinical Nursing, 13*(1), 65–74.

Trowell, J., & Etchegoyen, A. (2002). *The importance of fathers: A psychoanalytic re-evaluation. The new library of psychoanalysis*. Hove: Routledge.

Wilson, M., & Daly, M. (1995). The man who mistook his wife for a chattel. In, J.H. Barkow, L. Cosmides, J. Tooby (Eds.), *The Adapted Mind. Evolutionary psychology and the generation of culture*. 1992. New York, NY: Oxford University Press.

Winnicott, D. (1948). Pediatrics and psychiatry. *British Journal of Medical Psychology, 21*(4), 229.

Winnicott, D. W. (1964). *The child, the family and the outside environment*. Harmondsworth: Penguin.

Influence of childhood trauma on depression in the INDDEP study

Anna Lea Docter, Almut Zeeck, Jörn von Wietersheim and Heinz Weiss

Traumatic experiences during childhood have been shown to be associated with a higher risk for depressive disorders, more severe symptoms, higher rates of comorbidity, and poorer response to therapy. This study aims to further investigate these links in a clinical sample, focusing especially on therapeutic outcome. Data were collected in a large naturalistic study on inpatient and day hospital treatment of depression at the beginning, the end and after treatment, with this article being a secondary data analysis. Occurrence of childhood trauma, depressive and other symptoms and therapeutic results were compared using robust MANOVA, multiple regression, mixed ANOVA, and Spearman's correlation. Results provide support for a relationship between childhood trauma and depressive and general symptom severity, the age of onset of depression and the occurrence of personality disorders and somatic diagnoses. There was a significant reduction of depressive symptomatology after therapy. Patients with childhood trauma did not differ significantly from controls in their response to treatment. Clinicians should take the high probability of childhood trauma in depressive patients and the consequent risk of more severe symptoms into account when taking a history and consider adjusting treatment, even if the present data showed that patients generally benefitted from therapy.

Introduction

Epidemiological studies (Ferrari et al., 2013; Mathers, Fat, & Boerma, 2008; Wittchen et al., 2011) show that depressive disorders are repeatedly among the most frequent and most disabling psychiatric disorders with 12-month-prevalences for major depressive disorder (MDD) in European countries as high as 8.3% (Wittchen & Jacobi, 2005). Traumatic experiences during childhood occur in lifetime prevalences of up to 35% for physical and 9% for psychological abuse, 30% and 15% for sexual abuse in girls and boys, respectively, and 11.8% cumulative prevalence of neglect (Gilbert et al., 2009). These numbers showed significant variation depending on regions and types of assessment.

Psychodynamic concepts understand depression through theories revolving around experienced or imagined losses and processes of coping with them (Will, 2000), while cognitive behavioral ideas focus on learned helplessness or the lack of positive reinforcement. Biopsychological approaches have identified genes that predispose to the development of depression (Heils et al., 1996) and postulate neurological changes. Mostly, a multifactorial development is assumed.

Traumata during childhood frequently fall in the category of complex traumatization. Terr (1991) defined two trauma types, the first being caused by a singular event, while the second type follows repeated or continuous exposure to harmful events. Childhood traumas are often type II traumas. Furthermore, they frequently involve abuse within the family, thereby resulting in a relationship trauma (Ferenczi, 1931, 1949) which can influence attachment and identification processes or the experience of guilt. Other psychoanalytic ideas include the concept of cumulative trauma (Khan, 1974) with the experience of repeated lack of protection by the primary object. Childhood trauma can be differentiated by the categories of emotional and physical neglect and abuse, respectively, and sexual abuse (Krischer, Maya, & Sevecke, 2011). Theories about the impact of traumas focus on their meaning through and for relationships (Fonagy, 2005), on psychodynamic mechanisms (Fenichel, 1945), learned helplessness, or trauma memory (Ehlers & Clark, 2000; Foa & Rothbaum, 1998; Leuzinger-Bohleber, 2009). Some cognitive behavioral theories focus on characteristics of memory after trauma (e.g. little autobiographic integration and more pronounced associative learning), while psychodynamic theories try to integrate concepts like embodiment of memories and the reactivation of interaction patterns.

A connection between depression and childhood trauma has repeatedly been postulated and empirically shown: Trauma can be regarded as a risk factor for depression, but some theories also see depression as one subgroup of complex posttraumatic disorders (Laugharne, Lillee, & Janca, 2010; O'Donnell, Creamer, & Pattison, 2004; Seidler, 2013). Several of the aforementioned theories about either trauma or depression can be integrated in an attempt to understand these associations.

Various empirical studies have shown correlations of trauma and depression: The onset, severity, and therapeutic response of the latter are affected as well as its characteristics. This research has shown that individuals with traumatic childhood experiences show less secure attachment and more severe depressive symptoms (Styron & Janoff-Bulman, 1997), late therapeutic response (after 18 weeks of treatment) (Cropp, Zimmermann, & Streeck-Fischer, 2014) and a faster development of more depressive symptoms if a combination with dysfunctional cognitions and maladaptive coping occurs (Morris, Kouros, Fox, Rao, & Garber, 2014). Furthermore, it has been found that more depressive disorders emerge after childhood trauma, especially if genetic moderators lead to a strong association (Caspi et al.,

2003). Traumatic experiences also show associations with a higher risk, mostly for early onset depression, but also for depression in later life (Comijs et al., 2013) and a higher risk for chronic depressive disorders (Nanni, Uher, & Danese, 2012; Wiersma, Hovens, & van Oppen, 2009). Patients with childhood trauma also respond less to therapeutic interventions (Zlotnick, Ryan, Miller, & Keitner, 1995). Between a quarter and a third of traumatized children may develop a depressive episode by the end of their twenties (Gilbert et al., 2009). Depressive patients who have experienced sexual abuse during childhood had higher rates of comorbidity including axis-I- and axis-II-disorders (Zlotnick, Mattia, & Zimmerman, 2001). Differentiation with regard to trauma types and severity yield several results for associations with depression. One study found that emotional abuse showed the strongest association with depressive symptoms (Chapman et al., 2004), while another one showed that sexual abuse was also associated with depression (Andrews, Corry, Slade, Issakidis, & Swanston, 2004). Other findings showed that physical and emotional abuse and neglect were associated with the onset of depressive disorders (Norman et al., 2012) and that neglect and emotional abuse were most strongly associated with depression (Mandelli, Petrelli, & Serretti, 2015).

There is now a large number of meta-analyses, RCTs and large studies confirming the efficacy of psychotherapy, both cognitive behavioral and psychodynamic, in the treatment of depressive disorders (Butler, Chapman, Forman, & Beck, 2006; Dekker et al., 2014; Driessen et al., 2010; Fonagy et al., 2015; Huber & Klug, 2016; Jakobsen et al., 2007; Leichsenring, 2001).

Summarizing these findings, there is not only a general correlation between childhood trauma and the onset of depression, but the influence seems to be more specific. The characteristics of depression in patients who have experienced childhood trauma appear to be an earlier onset, more frequent chronicity and higher comorbidity. Furthermore, empirical research indicates a stronger association of emotional neglect and abuse with depressive symptoms than of other trauma types, at the same time being subject to a dose–effect relationship.

This study aims to assess childhood trauma rates in a clinical sample of patients that had to be hospitalized because of their depressive symptoms. It explores whether the kind or severity of childhood trauma is associated with the severity of depressive and other psychiatric symptoms. Furthermore, it aims to investigate therapeutic response, namely if patients with and without traumatic experiences show different responses to treatment when looking at the course of depressive symptoms. Comorbidities and specific symptoms are assessed and response to therapy is analyzed depending on the trauma history.

Hypotheses

The tested hypotheses are the following:

(1) The experience of childhood trauma is associated with more severe symptoms: groups of patients that differ in whether they have experienced childhood trauma also differ in the severity of their impairment

defined by several outcome measures: depressive symptoms, overall severity of psychological disorder, the age of onset of depression, additional somatic symptoms, and the number of comorbid personality disorders.

(2) Emotional neglect and abuse show the strongest association with depression.

(3) Patients with and without childhood trauma differ in their response to treatment, traumatized patients showing less symptom reduction at discharge and follow-up.

(4) Severe childhood trauma correlates with a lower level of psychic structure, which is conceptualized as a personality trait consisting of intrapsychic abilities concerning attachment and self-control, as well as being able to perceive and interact with self and others.

Methods

Setting

Data were generated in a multicentric naturalistic study on hospital and day hospital treatment in depression, the Inpatient and Day Hospital Treatment for Depression (INDDEP) study (Zeeck et al., 2015; Zeeck, Wietersheim, Weiss, Beutel, & Hartmann, 2013). Six hundred and four patients with a main diagnosis of a major depressive disorder, and at least moderate depression disorder (QIDS-C (see below) value >10) and an age of 18–65 years were assessed during four measure points: admission (T0), discharge (T1), and follow-up after three (T2) and twelve months (T3). The complete study design can be found in the study protocol (Zeeck et al., 2013). Patients underwent an intense multimodal treatment for depression in eight so-called psychosomatic hospitals in Germany, in either an in-patient or day hospital setting. The German health care system provides psychiatric and psychosomatic day hospital, in- and outpatient settings as common state-funded treatment options for mental disorders. Psychosomatic hospitals focus more on a psychotherapeutic approach while integrating psychopharmacological and somatic treatment. Representative for psychosomatic settings, treatment include group psychotherapy (symptom oriented and/or psychodynamic), individual psychotherapy with a frequency of one to two sessions per week, music, art, and body-oriented therapy and family sessions. Furthermore, patients have access to support by social workers, relaxation groups, educational groups, and sessions with the nursing team. Pharmacotherapy and medical care are also provided.

Measures

The information used in this study includes sociodemographic data, information about the hospital stay and data from the QIDS-C, SCL-90-R, CTQ, OPD-SQ,

SCID I and II as measures for depression, general psychiatric symptoms, trauma during childhood, psychic structure, and psychiatric diagnoses, respectively.

The clinician rating of the Quick Inventory of Depressive Symptomatology (QIDS-C) is based on the DSM IV criteria for depressive episodes and refers to the last seven days (Rush, Trivedi, & Ibrahim, 2003). Criterion validity has been shown by high correlations with other measures of depression, internal consistency is Cronbach's $\alpha = .85$.

The Symptom-Checklist (SCL-90-R) is a self-report questionnaire for physical and psychological symptoms during the last seven days. Internal consistency is $\alpha = .96$-.98, test–retest-reliability is $\alpha = .69$–.92, discriminant and convergent validity have also been shown (Franke & Derogatis, 2002).

The Childhood Trauma Questionnaire (CTQ) is a retrospective self-report instrument for trauma experienced during childhood and consists of five subscales: physical abuse and neglect, emotional abuse and neglect and sexual abuse (Krischer et al., 2011). A high internal consistency and an acceptable to excellent retest reliability have been shown for the CTQ. Established cut-offs (Negele, Kaufhold, Kallenbach, & Leuzinger-Bohleber, 2015; Walker, Unutzer, Rutter, et al., 1999) were used for the five subscales, each reaching a minimum value indicating relevant trauma in that dimension. These cut-offs were values of 10 for emotional abuse, 15 for emotional neglect and 8 for physical abuse, physical neglect and sexual abuse.

The Operationalized Psychodynamic Diagnostics Structure Questionnaire (OPD-SQ) is a self-report measure for psychic structure (Schauenburg, Dinger, & Komo-Lang, 2012). It refers to axis IV of the OPD (OPD Task Force, 2008), a descriptive diagnostic manual which is based on psychoanalytic concepts such as psychic structure, intrapsychic conflict, and transference. In this conceptualization, psychic structure is understood as a combination of capacities such as keeping boundaries, perception of self and other and self-control. An acceptable to good internal consistency has been shown for the OPD-SQ, validity is assumed based on the theoretical foundation as well as findings showing that patients with personality disorders have an overall lower psychic structure (Ehrenthal et al., 2012).

Diagnoses were given by experienced raters using the SCID I and II (Structured Clinical Interview for the Diagnostic and Statistical Manual of Mental Disorders (DSM-IV)), which shows good to excellent interrater reliability and acceptable to good test–retest-reliability for SCID II. Validity is given by the consistence with DSM criteria (Strauß, 2005).

Analysis

Data were analyzed using R (R Development Core Team, 2008), a statistical computing and graphics software.

The statistical methods used were robust MANOVA, multiple regression, mixed ANOVA, and Spearman's correlation. MANOVA (multivariate analysis of variance) analyzes associations between several variables and the dependent variable. Multiple regression tries to predict values of the dependent variable using several variables as predictors. Mixed ANOVA (analysis of variance) analyzes a combination of repeated measurements for one subject with comparisons between subjects. If sphericity is violated, Greenhouse–Geisser estimates are a conservative way of correcting for the violation. Bonferroni *post hoc* tests are used in the case of a significant ANOVA result to analyze which means differ significantly from one another.

Post hoc power tests using G*Power (Faul, Erdfelder, Buchner, & Lang, 2009; Faul, Erdfelder, Lang, & Buchner, 2007) showed sufficient power (>.8) for multiple regression and Spearman's correlation.

For the first hypothesis, an independent MANOVA was planned to analyze possible differences in several symptom measures depending on the existence of previous childhood trauma. Since testing for the preconditions for an independent MANOVA yielded negative results for the assumption of a multivariate normal distribution, a robust MANOVA was conducted. This was done following the method of Munzel and Brunner implemented in the mulrank()-function in R (Munzel & Brunner, 2000; Wilcox, 2005), which is based on ranking the data. Childhood trauma as measured in the CTQ was used as the independent variable. For this, the trauma subscales of the CTQ were dichotomized using established cut-offs (Negele et al., 2015; Walker et al., 1999) for the existence of relevant trauma. If the cut-off was reached in at least one subscale, the case was sorted into the trauma group. The QIDS-C total score, the global severity index of the SCL-90-R, the age of onset of depression, the number of somatic diagnoses (as diagnosed using the International Classification of Diseases (ICD-10)), and the number of personality disorders were used as dependent variables.

For the second hypothesis, preconditions for multiple regression (linearity, independence, equal variances, and normality) using the CTQ-subscales as predictors and the QIDS-C as dependent variable were fulfilled. A multiple regression was calculated to differentiate between the effects of different trauma types on the severity of depressive symptoms at admission using the lm()-function in R. The CTQ subscales were again dichotomized using cut-offs to assess if relevant trauma had occurred and were then used as independent variables. The total score of the QIDS-C was used as dependent variable.

To investigate effects of trauma on therapeutic results for the third hypothesis, a mixed ANOVA was conducted. To use the CTQ score as independent variable, the subscales were dichotomized and summed up following the steps used in the first hypothesis, resulting in a group with and a group without relevant trauma. The total score of the QIDS-C at T0 to T3 was used as dependent variable. Preconditions were fulfilled, the ezANOVA()-function of R was used and results were corrected for violation of sphericity using Greenhouse–Geisser estimates to

Table 1. Description of the study sample.

	Number	Percentage (%)
Sex		
Male	209	34.6
Female	395	65.4
Relationship		
Yes	275	45.5
No	329	54.5
Employed		
Yes	433	71.7
No	171	28.3
School Education		
Less than 10 years	294	48.7
At least 10 years	299	49.5

	Mean (SD)	Range
Age in years	43.1 (11.8)	19–65

adjust the degrees of freedom. The pairwise.t.test()-function was used to conduct Bonferroni *post hoc* tests.

For the fourth hypothesis investigating childhood trauma and psychic structure, the analysis contains only the subgroup to which the OPD-SF had also been administered (N = 260). A Spearman's correlation between childhood trauma measured by the total score of the CTQ and psychic structure measured by the total score of the OPD-SF was calculated using the cor.test()-function.

Results

An overview of the sociodemographic and symptom-associated data can be seen in Table 1. On average patients showed moderate depression (QIDS-C $m = 15.5$, SD = 3.1). For overall symptom severity, the GSI of the SCL-90-R showed $m = 1.43$, SD = .6.

About three-quarters of the patients in the study have suffered from childhood trauma, meaning that they have suffered traumatic experiences above the cut-off level in at least one CTQ subscale. The most frequent trauma types were emotional abuse, emotional neglect, and physical abuse (Table 2).

The robust MANOVA for the first hypothesis showed a significant main effect ($F = 4.96$, $p = 1.18e^{-13}$) of the experience of childhood trauma on the severity of depressive symptoms, overall symptom severity, age of onset of depression

Table 2. Depression, trauma, and comorbidity in the study sample.

	Mean (SD)	Range
Depression severity (QIDS-C)	15.5 (3.1)	10–25
Age at onset	32.8 (13.6)	5–61
Duration of current episode (weeks)	55.3 (70.1)	2–520
Number of previous episodes	3.3 (6.6)	1–135

	Number	Percentage (%)
Trauma types		
Emotional abuse	336	55.6
Emotional neglect	253	41.9
Sexual abuse	96	15.9
Physical abuse	179	29.6
Physical neglect	276	45.7
Trauma types experienced		
None	167	27.6
One	120	19.9
Two	93	15.4
Three	98	16.2
Four	90	14.9
Five	36	6.0

	Mean (SD)	Range
CTQ total score	54.9 (19.3)	28–124
Symptom severity (GSI)	1.43 (.60)	.16–3.39
Number of other axis-I diagnoses	1.0 (1.1)	0–7
Number of Axis-II diagnoses (PD)	.6 (.9)	0–5
Number of somatic diagnoses	1.1 (1.4)	0–5
Duration of therapy (days)	69.8 (29.8)	8–267

	Number	Percentage (%)
Setting		
Inpatient	301	49.8
Outpatient	303	50.2
Antidepressants at T3	287	47.5

Table 3. Statistical analyses – hypothesis 2.

	ΔR^2	*B*	SE *B*	*β*	*p*
Model	.02				<.001
Constant		15.14	.21		<.001
Emotional abuse		.03	.32	.01	.92
Physical abuse		−.49	.32	−.07	.13
Sexual abuse		.25	.37	.03	.49
Emotional neglect		.82	.35	.13*	.02
Physical neglect		.33	.31	.05	.29

and comorbidity including somatic diagnoses as well as personality disorders. Almost consistently the group with childhood trauma showed higher ranks for the outcome measures (lower ranks result for the age of onset). When differentiated by childhood trauma, the differences for depressive symptoms, psychiatric symptoms, and onset of depression were more pronounced than the differences in somatic diagnoses and personality disorders.

For the second hypothesis, the calculated multiple regression showed a small but significant prediction of depression severity by the model of the five trauma subscales, with emotional neglect having the main influence and being the only significant subscale. The additional predictive value of the other four subscales was close to zero when compared to a regression model using only emotional neglect as predictor. However, even the model using all five subscales explained only 2% of the dependent variable's variance (Table 3).

For the therapeutic response in the third hypothesis, the mixed ANOVA showed a significant main effect of the time of measurement, while not showing a significant main effect for traumatization or a significant interaction effect. In the Bonferroni *post hoc* tests, there were several significant differences in depression severity between time points: The time of admission differed significantly from all later measure points, time of discharge was significantly different from the first follow-up measure and the two follow-up measures also differed from one another (Table 4, Figure 1).

The calculation for the fourth hypothesis showed a significant ($p < .001$.), but small correlation of $r_s = .29$ between psychic structure and childhood trauma, a lower structural level being associated with more intense traumatization.

Discussion

Strengths and limitations of the study

In the INDDEP study, the data of a clinical sample were collected in a short amount of time creating a large data-set with few dropouts and missing data. The study's wide inclusion criteria resulted in good external validity, showing a high rate and

Table 4. Statistical analyses – hypothesis 3.

	df	*F*	*p*
Main effect (time)	2.87, 1158.67	317.09	<.001
Main effect (trauma)	1, 404	3.23	.073
Interaction effect	2.87, 1158.67	2.55	.057

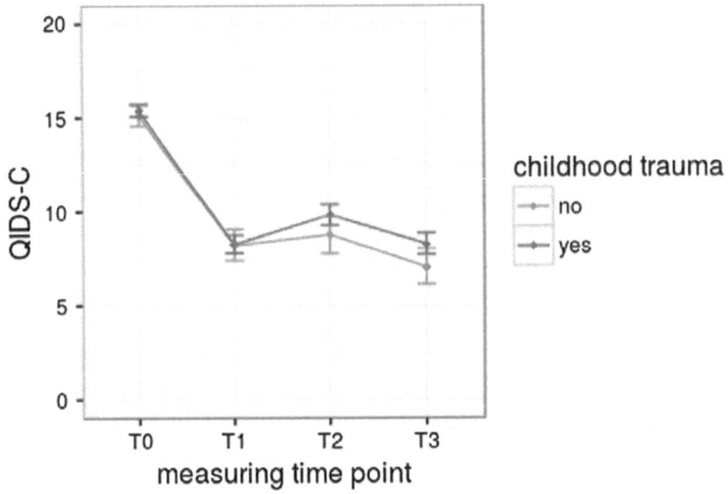

Figure 1. Course of therapeutic response.
Notes: Change in depressive symptoms over the course of treatment differentiated by experience of childhood trauma.

variety of comorbidities as is encountered in regular clinical work. The setting is representative for psychosomatic wards in Germany, a pilot study has ensured that possible setting differences do not influence the results (Zeeck, Hartmann et al., 2009; Zeeck, von Wietersheim et al., 2009) and the follow-up measure points allowed the assessment of the stability of therapeutic responses.

The clinical sample makes it impossible to investigate epidemiological questions and limits possible statements about the influences on the development of depressive symptoms. The relatively high impairment of patients with a QIDS value >10 and the requirement for intensive therapy probably limits the variance in other measures, especially rates of childhood trauma, which are markedly higher than in the general population. The limitation to Germany, German-speaking patients and the public health care system is a necessary practical requirement, but could lower the proportion of individuals with a very low socioeconomic status, who are less likely to enter a psychosomatic setting or have limited access to health care in general, a group which is also more often subject to traumatic experiences (Häuser, Schmutzer, Brähler, & Glaesmer, 2011).

The study was conducted as a naturalistic study and accordingly does not meet the criteria for a RCT design, therefore some of the therapeutic response could be attributable to other factors such as spontaneous remissions. In particular, it must be noted that the response to treatment cannot be attributed to one separate treatment module, but should be regarded as the result of the combined treatments in the day hospital consisting of several kinds of individual and group therapies, supported by a general psychodynamic understanding.

Measuring childhood trauma retrospectively has been challenged, however the CTQ has been shown to yield valid and stable results (Paivio, 2001; Wingenfeld et al., 2010).

Review of results

Trauma severity

The severity of childhood trauma was calculated by the number of CTQ subscales in which a cut-off was reached. Other approaches, such as using the total score, would be possible. We see the occurrence of several kinds of childhood trauma as the result of a potentially damaging trauma-facilitating family environment influencing personal development and the onset of psychopathology.

The calculated robust MANOVA limits the possible interpretations of the results, since it uses ranked data. However, a confirmation of the postulated connections can be deducted, as there seems to be a correlation between the number of experienced forms of childhood trauma and psychiatric, especially depressive symptoms and the age of onset of depression, which has been shown in previous studies (Chapman et al., 2004; Essau, Lewinsohn, Seeley, & Sasagawa, 2010; Klein et al., 2009; Moskvina et al., 2007; Norman et al., 2012; Withers, Tarasoff, & Stewart, 2013) and should be subject to further research.

Types of trauma

Although the hypothesis and previous results (Mandelli et al., 2015) are formally confirmed by the results of the multiple regression, the quantification shows this can be seen as a small tendency at best, with limited clinical significance. A future approach could be to investigate if the explained variance is higher if there is no limitation of the dependent variable by the inclusion criteria.

Response to therapy

The results of the mixed ANOVA showed a good therapeutic response in the reduction of depressive symptoms. As shown before (Dinger et al., 2015), depressive symptoms increased slightly after discharge to then decrease between the 3- and the 12-month-follow-up, which could be attributed to separation and adjustment processes (Pflichthofer, 2013; Rieber-Hunscha, 2007). The depressive scores never reach the level of that on admission to therapy, thereby indicating stable therapeutic results.

However, there is no significant effect of childhood trauma on therapeutic response in contrast to previous findings of patients with traumatization benefitting less or later from therapy (Cropp et al., 2014). One reason for this could be the duration of therapy, which was individually decided depending on the condition of the patient, so that patients who take more time to establish a good therapeutic relationship or to work through trauma-associated topics could stay in therapy for a longer amount of time. It is also possible that therapists adapted to the needs of their patients, focusing on trauma therapy when needed. When looking at the duration of therapy, the average variation of two days between groups with and without trauma should not be substantial. However, with an average duration of 70 days it could be possible that differences between groups decrease over time so that patients with childhood trauma benefit as well and show similarly stable therapeutic responses. When looking at the descriptive depiction of the results, the groups show similar scores for T0 and T1, but the scores of the group with traumatic experiences increase more at T2 and T3. There are, however, no significant differences here, which could indicate a stronger impact of separation on trauma victims. In this study, there has been no assessment of the proportion of patients with and without childhood trauma that proceed to undergo therapy in an outpatient setting. This question remains subject to further research.

The significant correlation can be seen as an indicator for an existing connection between childhood trauma and psychic structure. Psychic structure is conceptualized here as a psychological trait developing during early childhood, which can be affected by traumatic experiences and a negative family environment. Positive influences by external attachment figures as resilience factors are also possible, as well as modification in adulthood (Engle, Castle, & Menon, 1996; Stasch & Cierpka, 2014). The small correlation fits the idea of seeing psychic structure as a multidimensional construct.

Theoretical and practical implications

Findings and theories about the more frequent occurrence of depressive symptoms in people with traumatic experiences during childhood (Chapman et al., 2004) and influences of trauma types on specific symptom complexes (Mandelli et al., 2015; Norman et al., 2012; van Veen et al., 2013) are important for prevention and early intervention programs. To benefit from research in clinical daily work, it is necessary to identify characteristics of patients and derive opportunities and risks: which interventions and courses of treatment are helpful, which topics relevant, when is a longer duration of therapy necessary and which patients are prone to relapse? In the context of childhood trauma, general prevalences and severity of traumatization in different groups are relevant as well as their influence on the symptoms which require treatment, possible comorbidities, symptom characteristics, and the requirements for therapy which result from it.

The results of this study can be integrated well into previous findings, even if some of the results only hint at trends or lack large effect sizes.

Childhood trauma in patients is of significant importance in the daily work of clinical staff. More severe depressive and psychiatric symptoms in patients with traumatic experiences underline the importance of taking a reliable trauma history on patient admission. This can help to record risks such as suicidality (Sarchiapone, Carli, Cuomo, & Roy, 2007; Teicher & Samson, 2013) and plan psychotherapeutic interventions as well as pharmacotherapy, which can be less effective in traumatized patients (Klein et al., 2009).

Previous studies have shown selective influences of different trauma types on psychiatric symptom complexes, however the results of such studies are mixed. The results of this study point to a limited practical relevance of such differentiation, suggesting that an approach which differentiates less between the specific kind, number or intensity of trauma may be more relevant. It may be that a harmful family environment and absence of protective parental figures are a more significant influence on the development of symptoms than specific influence of the traumatizing events themselves.

The findings in this study contradict previous results (Nanni et al., 2012) in that no relevant differences were detected between the therapeutic response in patients with and without childhood trauma, possibly owing to the duration and intensity of therapy in a psychosomatic setting (12–16 h of individual and group therapy per week), which might facilitate establishing a therapeutic working relationship in patients regardless of the severity of trauma experienced. Overall, patients benefitted well from therapy with a stable reduction of depressive symptoms, thereby confirming findings of good therapeutic results in psychosomatic settings in previous studies (Zeeck et al., 2009).

Future studies should aim at further investigating some of these questions, namely the differential effects of trauma types, possible differences in therapeutic response if the duration of therapy is shorter, but also if and how personality traits and interpersonal relationships, which can be strongly affected by childhood trauma, change over the course of psychodynamic therapy. It is important to focus not only on manifest symptoms, but also on the mechanisms via which traumatic experiences lead to the development of psychiatric disorders.

Acknowledgments

The authors would like to thank the Heidehof Stiftung and all participating centers and research assistants, in particular: Sabine Hermann and Elvira Bozykaya (University of Freiburg), Jamie Knoblauch (University of Ulm), Anja Kidess (Robert-Bosch-Krankenhaus, Stuttgart), Johannes Becker-Pfaff (Bürgerhospital, Stuttgart), Caroline Linn (Fürst-Stirum-Klinikum, Bruchsal) and Antje Haselbacher (University of Mainz).

Disclosure statement

No potential conflict of interest was reported by the authors.

Funding

The INDDEP study is being funded by a grant from the Heidehof Stiftung GmbH Stuttgart.

References

Andrews, G., Corry, J., Slade, T., Issakidis, C., & Swanston, H. (2004). Child sexual abuse. In M. Ezzati, A. D. Lopez, A. A. Rodgers, & C. J. L. Murray, Eds., *Comparative quantification of health risks: Global and regional burden of disease attributable to selected major risk factors* (Vol. *2*, pp. 1851–1940). Geneva: World Health Organization.

Butler, A. C., Chapman, J. E., Forman, E. M., & Beck, A. T. (2006). The empirical status of cognitive-behavioral therapy: A review of meta-analyses. *Clinical Psychology Review, 26*(1), 17–31.

Caspi, A., Sugden, K., Moffitt, T. E., Taylor, A., Craig, I. W., Harrington, H., & Poulton, R. (2003). Influence of life stress on depression: Moderation by a polymorphism in the 5-HTT gene. *Science, 301*(5631), 386–389.

Chapman, D. P., Whitfield, C. L., Felitti, V. J., Dube, S. R., Edwards, V. J., & Anda, R. F. (2004). Adverse childhood experiences and the risk of depressive disorders in adulthood. *Journal of Affective Disorders, 82*(2), 217–225.

Comijs, H. C., van Exel, E., van der Mast, R. C., Paauw, A., Oude Voshaar, R., & Stek, M. L. (2013). Childhood abuse in late-life depression. *Journal of Affective Disorders, 147*(1–3), 241–246.

Cropp, C., Zimmermann, J., & Streeck-Fischer, A. (2014). Traumatisierungen in der Entwicklung – Unterschiedliche Verläufe stationärer Psychotherapie bei jugendlichen Patienten mit und ohne Traumatisierung [Developmental trauma – Differences between the course of inpatient treatment in adolescent patients with or without trauma history]. *Psychotherapie Psychosomatik Medizinische Psychologie, 68*(8), 328–335.

Dekker, J. J. M., Hendriksen, M., Kool, S., Bakker, L., Driessen, E., Jonghe, F. D., & Van, H. L (2014). Growing evidence for psychodynamic therapy for depression. *Contemporary Psychoanalysis, 50*(1–2), 131–155.

Dinger, U., Köhling, J., Klipsch, O., Ehrenthal, J. C., Nikendei, C., Herzog, W., & Schauenburg, H. (2015). Tagesklinische und stationäre Psychotherapie der Depression (DIP-D) – Sekundäre Erfolgsmaße und Katamneseergebnis einer randomisiert-kontrollierten Pilotstudie. [Day-clinic and inpatient psychotherapy of depression (DIP-D) – secondary outcomes and follow-up results of a randomized-controlled pilot trial]. *Psychotherapie Psychosomatik Medizinische Psychologie, 65*(7), 261–267.

Driessen, E., Cuijpers, P., de Maat, S. C., Abbass, A. A., de Jonghe, F., & Dekker, J. J. (2010). The efficacy of short-term psychodynamic psychotherapy for depression: A meta-analysis. *Clinical Psychology Review, 30*(1), 25–36.

Ehlers, A., & Clark, D. M. (2000). A cognitive model of posttraumatic stress disorder. *Behaviour Research and Therapy, 38*(4), 319–345.

Ehrenthal, J. C., Dinger, U., Horsch, L., Komo-Lang, M., Klinkerfuß, M., Grande, T., & Schauenburg, H. (2012). Der OPD-Strukturfragebogen (OPD-SF): Erste Ergebnisse zu Reliabilität und Validität. [The OPD structure questionnaire (OPD-SQ): First results on reliability and validity]. *Psychotherapie Psychosomatik Medizinische Psychologie, 62*(1), 25–32.

Engle, P. L., Castle, S., & Menon, P. (1996). Child development: Vulnerability and resilience. *Social Science & Medicine, 43*(5), 621–635.

Essau, C. A., Lewinsohn, P. M., Seeley, J. R., & Sasagawa, S. (2010). Gender differences in the developmental course of depression. *Journal of Affective Disorders, 127*(1–3), 185–190.

Faul, F., Erdfelder, E., Buchner, A., & Lang, A.-G. (2009). Statistical power analyses using G*Power 3.1: Tests for correlation and regression analyses. *Behavior Research Methods, 41*(4), 1149–1160.

Faul, F., Erdfelder, E., Lang, A.-G., & Buchner, A. (2007). G*Power 3: A flexible statistical power analysis program for the social, behavioral, and biomedical sciences. *Behavior Research Methods, 39*(2), 175–191.

Fenichel, O. (1945). *The psychoanalytic theory of neurosis*. New York, NY: Norton and Company.

Ferenczi, S. (1931). Child analysis in the analysis of adults. *The International Journal of Psychoanalysis, 12*, 468–482.

Ferenczi, S. (1949). Confusion of tongues between adults and the child. *The International Journal of Psychoanalysis, 30*, 225–230.

Ferrari, A. J., Charlson, F. J., Norman, R. E., Patten, S. B., Freedman, G., Murray, C. J., & Whiteford, H. A. (2013). Burden of depressive disorders by country, sex, age, and year: Findings from the global burden of disease study 2010. *PLoS Medicine, 10*(11), e1001547.

Foa, E. B., & Rothbaum, B. O. (1998). *Treating the trauma of rape*. New York, NY: Guilford Press.

Fonagy, P. (2005). *Affect regulation, mentalization, and the development of self.* New York, NY: Other Press.

Fonagy, P., Rost, F., Carlyle, J., McPherson, S., Thomas, R., Pasco Fearon, R., … Taylor, D. (2015). Pragmatic randomized controlled trial of long-term psychoanalytic psychotherapy for treatment-resistant depression: The Tavistock Adult Depression Study (TADS). *World Psychiatry, 14*(3), 312–321.

Franke, G. H., & Derogatis, L. R. (2002). *SCL-90-R*. Göttingen: Beltz.

Gilbert, R., Widom, C. S., Browne, K., Fergusson, D., Webb, E., & Janson, S. (2009). Burden and consequences of child maltreatment in high-income countries. *The Lancet, 373*(9657), 1368–1381.

Heils, A., Teufel, A., Petri, S., Stöber, G., Riederer, P., Bengel, D., & Lesch, K. P. (1996). Allelic variation of human serotonin transporter gene expression. *Journal of Neurochemistry, 66*(6), 2621–2624.

Huber, D., & Klug, G. (2016). Münchner psychotherapiestudie. [Munich psychotherapy study]. *Psychotherapeut, 61*(6), 462–467.

Häuser, W., Schmutzer, G., Brähler, E., & Glaesmer, H. (2011). Misshandlungen in Kindheit und Jugend: Ergebnisse einer Umfrage in einer repräsentativen Stichprobe der deutschen Bevölkerung. [Maltreatment in childhood and adolescence: Results from a survey of a representative sample of the German population]. *Deutsches Ärzteblatt International, 108*(17), 287–294.

Jakobsen, T., Rudolf, G., Brockmann, J., Eckert, J., Huber, D., Klug, G., & Leichsenring, F. (2007). Ergebnisse analytischer Langzeitpsychotherapien bei spezifischen psychischen Störungen: Verbesserungen in der Symptomatik und in interpersonellen Beziehungen. [Results of psychoanalytic long-term therapy in specific diagnostic groups: Improvernent in symptoms and interpersonal relationships]. *Zeitschrift für Psychosomatische Medizin und Psychotherapie, 53*(2), 87–110.

Khan, M. M. R. (1974). *The privacy of the self.* London: Hogarth Press.

Klein, D. N., Arnow, B. A., Barkin, J. L., Dowling, F., Kocsis, J. H., Leon, A. C., & Wisniewski, S. R. (2009). Early adversity in chronic depression: Clinical correlates and response to pharmacotherapy. *Depression and Anxiety, 26*(8), 701–710.

Krischer, K., Maya, K., & Sevecke. (2011). Klinisch-psychiatrische Ratingskalen für das Kindes- und Jugendalter. [Psychiatric rating scales for children and youth]. In C. Barkmann (Ed.), *Diagnostik für Klinik und Praxis* (pp. 133–137). Göttingen: Hofgrefe.

Laugharne, J., Lillee, A., & Janca, A. (2010). Role of psychological trauma in the cause and treatment of anxiety and depressive disorders. *Current Opinion in Psychiatry, 23*(1), 25–29.

Leichsenring, F. (2001). Comparative effects of short-term psychodynamic psychotherapy and cognitive-behavioral therapy in depression: A meta-analytic approach. *Clinical Psychology Review, 21*(3), 401–419.

Leuzinger-Bohleber, M. (2009). *Frühe Kindheit als Schicksal? Trauma, Embodiment, Soziale Desintegration. Psychoanalytische Perspektiven. [Early childhood as fate? Trauma, embodiment, social desintegration. Psychoanalytic perspectives].* Stuttgart: Kohlhammer.

Mandelli, L., Petrelli, C., & Serretti, A. (2015). The role of specific early trauma in adult depression: A meta-analysis of published literature. Childhood trauma and adult depression. *European Psychiatry, 30*(6), 665–680.

Mathers, C., Fat, D. M., & Boerma, J. T. (2008). *The global burden of disease: 2004 update*. Geneva: World Health Organization Press.

Morris, M. C., Kouros, C. D., Fox, K. R., Rao, U., & Garber, J. (2014). Interactive models of depression vulnerability: The role of childhood trauma, dysfunctional attitudes, and coping. *British Journal of Clinical Psychology, 53*(2), 245–263.

Moskvina, V., Farmer, A., Swainson, V., O'Leary, J., Gunasinghe, C., Owen, M., & Korszun, A. (2007). Interrelationship of childhood trauma, neuroticism, and depressive phenotype. *Depression and Anxiety, 24*(3), 163–168.

Munzel, U., & Brunner, E. (2000). Nonparametric tests in the unbalanced multivariate one-way design. *Biometrical Journal, 42*(7), 837–854.

Nanni, V., Uher, R., & Danese, A. (2012). childhood maltreatment predicts unfavorable course of illness and treatment outcome in depression: A meta-analysis. *American Journal of Psychiatry, 169*(2), 141–151.

Negele, A., Kaufhold, J., Kallenbach, L., & Leuzinger-Bohleber, M. (2015). Childhood Trauma and Its Relation to Chronic Depression in Adulthood. *Depression Research and Treatment, 2015*(5), 1–11.

Norman, R. E., Byambaa, M., De, R., Butchart, A., Scott, J., & Vos, T. (2012). The long-term health consequences of child physical abuse, emotional abuse, and neglect: A systematic review and meta-analysis. *PLoS Medicine, 9*(11), 1–31.

O'Donnell, M. L., Creamer, M., & Pattison, P. (2004, August). Posttraumatic stress disorder and depression following trauma: Understanding comorbidity. *American Journal of Psychiatry, 161*(8), 1390–1396.

OPD Task Force (Ed.). (2008). *Operationalized psychodynamic diagnosis OPD-2*. Göttingen u.a.: Hogrefe.

Paivio, S. C. (2001). Stability of retrospective self-reports of child abuse and neglect before and after therapy for child abuse issues. *Child Abuse & Neglect, 25*(8), 1053–1068.

Pflichthofer, D. (2013). The end of the analysis and the postanalytical relationship. *Forum der Psychoanalyse, 29*(2), 201–222.

R Development Core Team (2008). *R: A language and environment for statistical computing*. Vienna: R Foundation for Statistical Computing.

Rieber-Hunscha, I. (2007). Wann ist zu Ende therapiert? [When is therapy done?]. *PiD – Psychotherapie im Dialog, 8*(2), 108–116.

Rush, A. J., Trivedi, M. H., & Ibrahim, H. M. (2003). The 16-Item quick inventory of depressive symptomatology (QIDS), clinician rating (QIDS-C), and self-report (QIDS-SR): A psychometric evaluation in patients with chronic major depression. *Biological Psychiatry, 54*(5), 573–583.

Sarchiapone, M., Carli, V., Cuomo, C., & Roy, A. (2007). Childhood trauma and suicide attempts in patients with unipolar depression. *Depression and Anxiety, 24*(4), 268–272.
Schauenburg, H., Dinger, U., & Komo-Lang, M. (2012). Der OPD-Strukturfragebogen (OPD-SF). [The OPD structure questionnaire (OPD-SQ)]. In S. Doering & A. Buchheim (Eds.), *Handbuch der Strukturdiagnostik* (pp. 284–307). Stuttgart: Schattauer.
Seidler, G. H. (2013). *Psychotraumatologie* [Psychotraumatology]. Stuttgart: Kohlhammer.
Stasch, M., & Cierpka, M. (2014). *Operationalisierte psychodynamische Diagnostik OPD-2* [Operationalized psychodynamic diagnostics OPD-2]. Bern: Huber.
Strauß, B. (2005). *Klinische Interviews und Ratingskalen* [Clinical interviews and rating scales]. Göttingen u.a.: Hogrefe.
Styron, T., & Janoff-Bulman, R. (1997). Childhood attachment and abuse: Long-term effects on adult attachment, depression, and conflict resolution. *Child Abuse & Neglect, 21*(10), 1015–1023.
Teicher, M. H., & Samson, J. A. (2013). Childhood maltreatment and psychopathology: A case for ecophenotypic variants as clinically and neurobiologically distinct subtypes. *American Journal of Psychiatry, 170*(10), 1114–1133.
Terr, L. C. (1991). Childhood traumas: An outline and overview. *The American Journal of Psychiatry, 148*(1), 10–20.
van Veen, T., Wardenaar, K., Carlier, I., Spinhoven, P., Penninx, B., & Zitman, F. (2013). Are childhood and adult life adversities differentially associated with specific symptom dimensions of depression and anxiety? Testing the tripartite model. *Journal of Affective Disorders, 146*(2), 238–245.
Walker, E., Unutzer, J., Rutter, C., Gelfand, A., Saunders, K., Von Korff, M., Koss, M. P., Katon, W. (1999). Costs of Health Care Use by Women HMO Members With a History of Childhood Abuse and Neglect. *Archives of General Psychiatry, 56*(7), 609–613.
Wiersma, J. E., Hovens, J. G. F. M., & van Oppen, P. (2009). The importance of childhood trauma and childhood life events for chronicity of depression in adults. *Journal of Clinical Psychiatry, 70*(7), 983–989.
Wilcox, R. R. (2005). *Introduction to robust estimation and hypothesis testing*. Amsterdam: Elsevier.
Will, H. (2000). *Depression*. Stuttgart: Kohlhammer.
Wingenfeld, K., Spitzer, C., Mensebach, C., Grabe, H. J., Hill, A., Gast, U., & Driessen, M. (2010). Die deutsche Version des Childhood Trauma Questionnaire (CTQ): Erste Befunde zu den psychometrischen Kennwerten. [The German version of the Childhood Trauma Questionnaire (CTQ): Preliminary psychometric properties]. *Psychotherapie Psychosomatik Medizinische Psychologie, 60*(11), 442–450.
Withers, A. C., Tarasoff, J. M., & Stewart, J. W. (2013). Is depression with atypical features associated with trauma history? *Journal of Clinical Psychiatry, 74*(5), 500–506.
Wittchen, H.-U., & Jacobi, F. (2005). Size and burden of mental disorders in Europe—A critical review and appraisal of 27 studies. *European Neuropsychopharmacology, 15*(4), 357–376.
Wittchen, H. U., Jacobi, F., Rehm, J., Gustavsson, A., Svensson, M., Jönsson, B., & Steinhausen, H.-C. (2011). The size and burden of mental disorders and other disorders of the brain in Europe 2010. *European Neuropsychopharmacology, 21*(9), 655–679.
Zeeck, A., Hartmann, A., Küchenhoff, J., Weiss, H., Sammet, I., Gaus, E., … Wietersheim, J. V. (2009). Differenzielle indikationsstellung stationärer und tagesklinischer psychotherapie: Die DINSTAP-studie [Differential indication of inpatient and day clinic treatment in psychosomatics]. *Psychotherapie Psychosomatik Medizinische Psychologie, 59*, (09/10), 354–363.

Zeeck, A., von Wietersheim, J., Hartmann, A., Einsele, S., Weiss, H., Sammet, I., & Küchenhoff, J. (2009). Inpatient or day clinic treatment? Results of a multi-site-study. *GMS Psycho-Social-Medicine, 6*, 1–11.

Zeeck, A., von Wietersheim, J., Weiß, H., Eduard Scheidt, C., Völker, A, Helesic, A., & Hartmann, A. (2015). Symptom course in inpatient and day clinic treatment of depression: Results from the INDDEP-Study. *Journal of Affective Disorders, 187*, 35–44.

Zeeck, A., Wietersheim, J. V., Weiss, H., Beutel, M., & Hartmann, A. (2013). The INDDEP study: Inpatient and day hospital treatment for depression – Symptom course and predictors of change. *BMC Psychiatry, 13*(1), 1–7.

Zlotnick, C., Mattia, J., & Zimmerman, M. (2001). Clinical features of survivors of sexual abuse with major depression. *Child Abuse & Neglect, 25*(3), 357–367.

Zlotnick, C., Ryan, C. E., Miller, I. W., & Keitner, G. I. (1995). Childhood abuse and recovery from major depression. *Child Abuse & Neglect, 19*(12), 1513–1516.

Epilogue: How Shall We Defeat the 6th Giant Now?

We were not to know in 2017, when we planned a special Journal edition, which our publishers agreed to bring together in a book format in 2020, that NICE's new depression guideline itself would not be finished. NICE's Committee Chair, Professor Kapur, joked that several of our members had started a family and seen their children into primary school whilst we were still labouring away evaluating the evidence base. The new guideline, we were told, would not see the light of day until 2021. Our task – a vast network meta-analysis – had become a huge and complex undertaking. In fact, McPherson et al., in persisting with their criticisms of our earlier efforts (Chapter 1) and succeeding in meeting directly with NICE, were primarily responsible for an unprecedented U-turn by the committee. In late 2019, it was announced by NICE that consultation on a 3rd draft guideline would take place. Having previously defended its methodology NICE had now agreed to a re-analysis of the evidence to address the admitted shortcomings of its earlier evaluations. As a member of NICE's committee myself I am precluded from further comment other than to observe that I was pleased at this outcome. It also marks a welcome watershed within our own discipline.

The pioneering empirical research of George Brown and Tirril Harris in the 1970s (Brown and Harris, 1978) first helped to establish a clear causal connection between loss of close, interpersonal support, often through early bereavement or economic migration, and the fragility of those attachment bonds that were 'left behind', for generations of women, living with and suffering depression in deprived communities in Camberwell, South London. Two decades later, working as a counsellor in a GP Practice on Coldharbour Lane, I saw for myself the impact of ongoing social adversity on a new generation of families. So, when Professor Lord Richard Layard's *Depression Report* (2005) led to setting up a first, universal access, free-at-point-of-need national talking therapies service, for me to be invited to give a speech at the Maudsley Hospital, South London, to welcome the Secretary of State Rt. Hon. Alan Johnson MP to launch IAPT, felt like a privilege and a moment of genuine change.

What I said on that occasion was that Depression could be seen as a 6th Giant Evil, alongside the 5 Giant Social Evils that Beveridge had made it the mission of the Welfare State to aim to defeat: Want, Disease, Squalor, Ignorance and Idleness. In that year, the World Health Organisation was predicting depression would become the single greatest disease burden by 2020 (WHO, 2008). But the essential point for us, I said, was to see beyond the external facts of a person's situation, not to deny these needs, but to address their complex, often invisible connection with an individual's suffering of depression. Unless we helped people's mental well-being, Beveridge's welfare vision, to support people back on their feet, would fail. What happened? Sadly, the Psychiatric Morbidity Survey (McManus et al, 2016) showed the burden of depression grew over the next decade: anti-depressant prescriptions rose especially steeply in those parts of the country where social deprivation had got worse. Increased self-harm and rising rates of suicide further underlined our failure. Yet in 2020 well over 1 million NHS patients in IAPT will be offered what NICE tells us are our two most effective treatments with the 'strongest evidence' namely Cognitive Behavioural Therapy (CBT), alongside or instead of anti-depressants. Even mission control at NHS England HQ was admitting 'we have a problem'.

The thread that runs through our chapters in this volume points to the solution hiding in plain sight ever since the work of Brown and Harris in the 1970s: depression's social origins.

By speaking up for the importance of these aspects of a person's depression when we offer our psychotherapeutic interventions we are now, perhaps, edging towards a new paradigm.

Nobody has set out this challenge so well as Andrew Solomon (2001), whose book, *The Noonday Demon: An Anatomy of Depression*, goes straight to the heart of society's angst:

> Depression is the flaw in love. To be creatures who love, we must be creatures who can despair at what we lose, and depression is the mechanism of that despair. When it comes, it degrades one's self and ultimately eclipses the capacity to give or receive affection. It is the aloneness within us made manifest, and it destroys not only connection to others but also the ability to be peacefully alone with oneself. (p. 15)

Solomon is part of a growing trend towards sufferers publishing first-hand experiences of illness in the form of Depression Memoirs (Radden & Varga, 2013). This trend is spurred on by campaigns to reduce long-standing stigma surrounding mental illness. Public figures such as Alastair Campbell and Stephen Fry have become ambassadors for these movements. The Young Royals, Princes William and Harry, together with Kate and Meghan, have come out bravely to continue what they see as the legacy of Princess Diana, whose struggles with her own mental health were cruelly pilloried by the media who hounded her during the 1990s.

It is beyond my scope here to review how this diverse literature and new level of public awareness has significance for our clinical understanding of depression. But I want to try to draw out some of its *potential* implications.

As noted by Jennifer Radden and Somogy Varga, and hence underlining the importance of Matthew Ratcliffe's work here (Chapter 2):

> These personal accounts have entered public discourse with the simultaneous decline in medical authority... A new vocabulary has been provided for personal narratives of illness by non-experts, giving voice to the experience of being ill, and focusing on the whole person often ignored in the medical sphere ...(p. 99–100)

In Linda Gask's (2015) memoir, *The Other Side of Silence,* these different perspectives are brought together. Gask writes as a Consultant Psychiatrist in the NHS, a highly respected academic who served as an Expert Adviser on NICE's guideline for Common Mental Health Disorders (NICE, CG 123, 2011), and a 'person who gets depressed' (p. 14):

> This is who I am. I cope most of the time; I am well for months, sometimes even for more than a year, but there are recurring periods in my life when the world seems a darker, more hostile and unforgiving place. (p. 14)

In her honest and reflective book, Gask describes the origins of this lifelong vulnerability to depression in her own case. Her mother was aged 12 when her own mother, Gask's grandmother, collapsed and died when they were out together in the street. The eldest of three children, with two younger brothers, Gask's middle brother, Alan, struggled throughout their childhood and was eventually diagnosed with OCD (obsessive compulsive disorder).

Together with the effort of supporting the family financially, Alan's difficulties put a strain on their father's relationship with their mother and the children. Her mother took Valium for anxiety, prescribed by the family GP; her father eventually seemed to become defeated by life and retreated to his bed, not able to get up for work for days at a time. Gask reflects:

> ... my family never really provided a safe, emotionally secure base for me to grow up and learn how to explore the world with confidence. (p. 25). She emphasises:
>
> The problem is that when you are caught deep in the jaws of depression, recapturing a sense of hope seems almost unimaginable. [Depression] colours the way we see our lives and clouds our judgement, not only about others but most particularly about ourselves. It is hard to think **positively**, as others often insist, when you consider yourself to be completely worthless. (p. 9–10)

In her conclusion to her memoir Gask makes clear she has benefited from talking therapies and anti-depressant medication as treatments and that 'each of these methods ... has played an important role' (p. 255). However, it is the interpersonal element that is key:

> ... each person has a different story to tell about their misery, and there are many different reasons why they have become depressed. Their life problems

> … are not simple but complex; they are intertwined with the other realities of the human condition: our vulnerability, fears, losses, wounds, the need to be loved, the pain of loneliness, the difficulty in trusting others, the problems in our past and unresolved grief. It's impossible to really help a person who is depressed without acknowledging and addressing these experiences. This is why medication on its own is never the answer (p. 255). Similarly, we can add, as Gask stresses, it is also why computerised CBT for many people should **not** be the first answer to treat a person's depression.

Yet we face a problem of unmet need for treatment of depression on a scale we have yet fully to grapple with. For this reason, although I have changed my view about IAPT (Clarke, forthcoming) and we made mistakes in design as well as implementation, I am not one of those who advocates throwing out the baby with the bathwater (Dalal, 2018; Jackson and Rizq, 2019). CBT and medication, in NICE's next guideline, will still be part of the answer if not, for sure, the whole. And the case for including *brief* psychodynamic therapy as standard in IAPT's offer, e.g. Dynamic Interpersonal Therapy (DIT; Chapters 3 and 5), has now been further strengthened by recent publication of its Randomised Controlled Trial (RCT; Fonagy et al, 2019):

> As IAPT services offer psychodynamic therapy, its efficacy in real-world settings is highly relevant to patients, therapists, and the healthcare system. Evidence for the efficacy of psychodynamic therapy for common mental disorders is available (Leichsenring et al., 2015), but this study is the first to demonstrate DIT's effectiveness in primary care. Encouraging remission rates were obtained, particularly given the severity of depression in the sample and the low recovery rate in the LIT* condition (p. 9). *LIT = low intensity therapies, such as computerised CBT.

From this RCT the headline implications for practice were (i) *The DIT and CBT arms showed equivalence on most outcomes* and (ii) *DIT delivered in a primary care setting is superior to LIT [low intensity therapy]* (p. 1). The trial sites were in Newham and Tower Hamlets, East London, so DIT proved itself in areas of social deprivation. In IAPT's 'set menu' DIT should now be implemented at scale, ideally as a first-line option whenever patient preference or presenting history indicates. For this question, an empirical one, we must defend the view that RCTs are not the only way to show causality: their yield to date does not tell us if one treatment will be better *for this patient* than another; we rely on expert clinical judgement.

The evidence-based case study by Tohar Dolev and her colleagues (Chapter 4) shows how we *can* generate useful knowledge about why a brief psychodynamic therapy worked well for one patient, but not the other. There is a resurgence of interest in single case studies (McLeod and Elliott, 2011). It is too soon to say if they will find a place in NICE's manual for evaluating evidence (Clarke & Stiles 2018). Likewise, the findings from the study by Anna Docter and her colleagues (Chapter 7) about the influence of childhood trauma on later life depression are a valuable addition to what we know from epidemiological research. At some point in time prognosis and treatment choice in depression will eventually be more personalised and informed by such evidence. But as yet there is no agreement on how to combine or synthesise 'observational facts'. At best we rely on what my colleague Nancy Cartwright calls 'artful modelling' (Cartwright, 2019). Our aim should be no less scientific for that and, on the contrary, it is how we can aspire to rigour and avoid the mistake we made – in my view – in IAPT's design: we adopted an over-simplified algorithm for depression from NICE's 2009 guideline, notwithstanding the caution we had flagged for *its* limited evidence (NICE, 2009, p. 128). At the start of IAPT the then Chair of NICE, Sir Michael Rawlins (2008), used his Harveian Oration *De Testimonio* to argue that we over-relied on RCTs. He was right.

In sum, NICE's Depression Guideline Committee is faced with a terrain of evidence that is vast and uncertain, with limited navigation tools for finding its way towards clear recommendations, conscious of heavy responsibility, not least for carrying with it a fragile trust and support across a now fragmented discipline, as well as for doing right by patients.

The chapters in this book do not report directly the results of any new RCTs for depression. Instead, they offer a contribution of a different kind. We can hope that whether or not they feature in the deliberations of NICE's committee, they do nevertheless represent as well as demonstrate the ongoing vitality and relevance of contemporary psychodynamic interventions. And whilst we must wait to see what the next NICE Guideline for Depression does in the end recommend, this Epilogue is also an opportunity to reflect on what we have learned since the previous guideline in 2009. Because the plain truth here is that none of our treatments *on their own* – possibly altogether – can (or even should?) defeat the many forms that depression manifests today. For if depression is indeed 'the flaw in love' it is also the reminder we must stop and take the time to find new ways to reconnect. This relates to the reason we have focused on depression in men in several chapters (Chapters 4, 5 and 6).

With regard to men with depression our intention was not primarily to highlight how they are a neglected group often in terms of NHS mental health services, though that fact is true (Bjerkeset et al, 2008). Happily, here we can report we are already making progress. As well as raising public awareness through recent anti-stigma campaigns using footballers talking about their own depression, stressing the need for men to feel able to ask for help, we are also actively engaged with NHS England to help staff in perinatal mental health services work effectively also with new fathers using brief, psychodynamic interventions. More fundamentally, though, our argument throughout this book calls for a different kind of rebalancing altogether. Our wish to return to the questions asked by Brown and Harris of their research participants in deprived parts of 1970s South London, through a lens on how these questions can be framed also for helping men, is more properly about the need to re-think our approach towards the whole idea about awareness raising, stigma and prevention.

In a book that is highly critical of the NICE/IAPT axis of evidence-based practice, the eminent sociologist, Nikolas Rose (2019), points to the difficulty of the real problem with prevention:

> Paradoxically, the belief in maximising virtue through entry into wage labour and the constraints on future conduct imposed by the need to secure one's employment career were being extolled at the very moment when that image of secure work was already becoming a thing of the past, with its belief of a universal and timeless pattern of life – the move from the disciplines of the family through those of schooling to those of a job for life, followed by a brief retirement and then death … all these and more now largely exist as images in our rear view mirror, already coloured in the sepia tones of nostalgia, their own inequities and injustices rapidly fading from memory. (p. vii)

By returning to those first-person Depression Memoirs, I have argued, we can begin at least to get a glimpse of the many ways that at one moment our enemy is a Behemoth, bestriding and wreaking particular havoc on those areas and populations left behind by austerity, whilst at another it can now shift shape in the form of a Leviathan, whose all-encompassing embrace in the seas that surrounds us can erode and batter our national morale post-Brexit. A prevention agenda to unravel the *intersection* of stigma with depression across our life course, and all parts of society, must follow the pioneering work done by Brown and Harris, as well as explore its causal links between income inequality and higher prevalence (Pickett and Wilkinson, 2010). Unless we understand better *how* presentations of stigma and depression manifest and interact, as well as *that* they manifest in some groups in growing numbers (Fink et al 2016), we will not know how best to intervene both early, promptly and late. Depression affects us all sooner or later, directly or indirectly. Preventing it from becoming a disabling, even deadly, illness continues to represent a major public mental health challenge for now and for the foreseeable future (Kousoulis and Goldie, 2017; 2018; Kousoulis, 2019).

Finally, then, I would like to describe some encouraging findings from a pilot project in Greater Manchester called *Working Well.* This speaks directly to the social and interpersonal origins of depression. When Lord Layard and myself sold the idea of IAPT to the Treasury in 2007, we made three promises, which I touch on in my introduction: (i) to increase access to talking therapies, (ii) to reduce the burden of depression and anxiety and (iii) to implement a sustainable model for scaling up these services by ensuring that savings could be re-invested from supporting people with chronic depression on incapacity benefits to return to work. We got the balance wrong. By adhering to NICE's 2009 stepped care algorithm, over-rigidly, the priority for the new IAPT services became more and more driven by access and waiting time targets. As a consequence of its misguided efforts to increase so-called 'productivity', NHS England made it more difficult for those on the frontline to help anyone whose needs were multiple, many-faceted, long-standing, acute and recurrent, or all at the same time.

In 2010, then, under the new Coalition government, I was asked to help Lord Freud at the Department for Work and Pensions (DWP). The providers of DWP's Work Programme were encountering large numbers of clients for employment support needing help for depression, in addition to support for returning to work. It made sense to try to join them up with IAPT. Lord Freud, as Minister for Welfare Reform, and Norman Lamb MP, then the Minister with responsibility for mental health, were persuaded to commission an independent review of evidence for a more integrated approach they could jointly promote (Van Stolk et al, 2014).

Based on RAND Europe's findings, and with the opportunity of regional devolution, Greater Manchester then invited me to help them design a new model that started at the other end from IAPT by targeting people on incapacity benefits with chronic and recurrent depression. Using what we knew about why IAPT had not worked for this group of patients we designed in some key features for *Working Well* that were different. Our programme did not adopt an algorithm based around a first-line offer of brief CBT; instead, it was a more personalised approach in which each client could engage with a wide range of support options for up to 2 years, with a further year of in-work support. It is important to note that whilst our design differed from IAPT in this way, all the talking therapies for depression in *Working Well* were those recommended in NICE's 2009 guideline. Setting ourselves an ambitious target of 20% 'real recovery', defined as *a capacity for sustained employment (over 12 months),* we persuaded the Cabinet Office and European Social Fund to give us a total funding of £10M.

In the words of Andy Burnham, the elected Mayor of Greater Manchester: *The success story that is Working Well sets our city region apart from the rest of the country.* (GMCA, 2018).

An independent evaluation found that Working Well achieved its ambitious target of getting 20% of its clients into stable employment for 52 weeks or more. How did it happen? The quantitative series of evaluations told us *whom* Working Well had worked for (and whom not). A more qualitative evaluation also explored *how and why* Working Well had worked (and how and why not). By using a realist evaluation methodology, rather than an RCT design, we were also able to find out about *Working Well's* limitations at its developmental stage (Deaton and Cartwright, 2017; Duncan et al, 2018). Our theory of change was that a Key worker role as the central point of contact for clients was best placed to facilitate an integrated, personalised schedule of support. This involved deploying employment support with mental health interventions in the right sequence and best combination for each client. We needed to test whether our assumptions about how Working Well might work, derived from designing in the key enabling factors identified in the joint evidence review, such as a common outcomes framework across employment support and mental health providers, could be made to work as expected in practice. For example, if an important task for the Key worker role was to help the client navigate their way to the right intervention for them, at the time they needed it, would the full menu of those options be made available for access?

What we learnt was that Working Well worked for some clients better than for others, and that where it didn't work, tended to be those clients who were older, were less qualified and had been out of work for longer, compared to those who did better who were younger, more qualified and with recent work experience. We also learnt that clients with previous convictions, or with substance and alcohol misuse problems, and more severe and complex mental and physical health issues, were those who proved especially challenging to help.

More surprising, though, was what we found out about our theory of change and the vital task around which the success of Working Well hinged: the Key worker role. We knew from experience in developing a new role in IAPT, the Psychological Wellbeing Practitioner role, we would encounter barriers to embedding this alongside existing roles (Turpin et al, 2009).

The research literature pointed us to established and traditional disciplines being protective in relation to any newcomers: *A culture of protecting professional and organisational identities is one of the most prominent barriers to new ways of working, especially where established skills and roles are reconfigured* (Gilburt, 2016). In the context of mental health IAPT itself was generally seen as disruptive by the established disciplines of Psychiatry and Clinical Psychology. For Working Well, we reasoned, the inclusion of *all* new roles across the Talking Therapies team, as well as Key worker teams, should result in *less* protectionism. We still expected integrated working would be a challenge in other respects, but less so in this.

Initially our findings confirmed what we had expected, and in some ways it remained true that integration proved most difficult at the level of meetings between the managers of the different providers, where their performance against outcomes targets would be discussed. Even here, however, we were taken aback by the extent of what appeared to be a breakdown in communication between the mental health service managers and other managers: 'They won't even talk to each other', we were told by commissioners. Indeed, reflecting on this, Working Well's programme commissioners felt it was mental health managers who would become especially defensive whenever problems with integrated ways of working came up. Our own experience as evaluators, admittedly coming from a background of expertise in mental health ourselves, did not bear this out. Nor was it clear why mental health managers would have felt defensive with regard to their own performance, since the results they were achieving with Working Well clients, whose profile was considerably more complex than in a typical IAPT service, showed consistently higher recovery rates than IAPT national averages.

It was through our close investigation of the Key worker role that we began to develop an understanding of how these barriers to communication were occurring and, importantly, find a way to help the different teams working directly with the clients to overcome them. We designed a series of Focus groups where the teams met with us to reflect on their roles. Key workers would meet with us first in their own team, as would Talking Therapists, and we would listen to each team's explanation about what was working successfully with their clients, and what wasn't, and then check back with them having picked up discrepancies between the various teams in their different accounts about the same issues with their client work, as to whether we had understood *their* version of what happened correctly. Then we held a further series of Focus groups where Key workers from different teams and Talking Therapists would meet together in the same Focus group discussion. This gave us an opportunity to encourage them to consider explanations for what happened with clients, in particular for what was not working so well with clients, other than their own account. Time and again the pattern that emerged was the dominance of those causal explanations put forward by the Talking Therapists, and deference of Key workers to their greater expertise.

I cannot do justice here to the rich material these Focus groups generated for our analysis. To describe how the process of evaluation evolved as a kind of action research, in which the different teams eventually found a way to listen to each other's perspectives without overt or more subtle forms of smothering of the *non-expert* accounts, does not really capture the complexity of what took place. In the view of the teams themselves, and their managers and commissioners, the value of this reflective space with each other was demonstrated over time through a capacity for mutual problem-solving and more effective joint working. Likewise, with clients, the Focus groups stimulated impromptu joint sessions, where client, Key worker and Talking Therapist would sit down all three together. Significant gains were seen, and intractable barriers to return to work and improved mental health were overcome.

Due to its impressive outcomes Working Well has already been scaled up in Greater Manchester. If it replicates its early success it may be taken up elsewhere. The key aspect of Working Well's success I have tried to convey here was how fragile and uncertain this was.

The last words should go to Andrew Solomon:

> Let us make no bones about it: We do not really know what causes depression. We do not really know what constitutes depression. We do not really know why certain treatments may be effective for depression. We do not know how depression made it through the evolutionary process. We do not know why one person gets a depression from circumstances that do not trouble another. (p. 29)

References

Bjerkeset, O. et al. (2008). Gender differences in the association of mixed anxiety and depression with suicide. *British Journal of Psychiatry 192(6)* pp. 474–5.

Brown, G.W. & Harris, T. (1978). *Social origins of depression: a study of psychiatric disorder in women.* London: Tavistock.

Cartwright, N. (2019). *Nature, the Artful Modeler. Lectures on Laws, Science, How Nature Arranges the World and How We Can Arrange It Better.* Chicago: Open Court.

Clarke, J.C. (forthcoming). If not a Tsunami of CBT, then what? The debate about NHS psychotherapy services in the age of Mc-IAPT. *British Journal of Psychotherapy.*

Clarke, J. C. & Stiles, W.B. (2018). Using model case studies experimentally to predict structural change in psychotherapy: can we theorise change mechanisms and trace causal processes to predict what will work for whom? Unpubl. Workshop, Institute of Advanced Study, Durham University, 6th November.

Deaton and Cartwright (2018) Understanding and misunderstanding randomized controlled trials *Social Science & Medicine* 210, 2–21.

Duncan et al (2018) A realist approach to the evaluation of complex mental health interventions *British Journal of Psychiatry* 213, 451–453.

Dalal, F. (2018). *CBT: The Cognitive Behavioural Tsunami. Managerialism, Politics and the Corruptions of Science* Abingdon, Oxon: Routledge.

Fink, E., Patalay, P., Sharpe, H., et al. (2015) Mental Health Difficulties in Early Adolescence: A Comparison of Two Cross-Sectional Studies in England From 2009 to 2014. The Journal of Adolescent Health: Official Publication of the Society for Adolescent Medicine. *56(5)* (pp. 502–507).

Fonagy P et al (2019). Dynamic interpersonal therapy for moderate to severe depression: a pilot randomized controlled and feasibility trial. *Psychological Medicine 1–10.* https://doi.org/10.1017/ S0033291719000928.

Gask, L. (2015). *The Other Side of Silence. A Psychiatrist's Memoir of Depression.* Chichester: Vie Books.

Gilburt (2016) *Supporting integration through new roles and working across boundaries.* London: Kings Fund.

GMCA (2018) *Working Well Annual Report* Greater Manchester Combined Authority.

Jackson, C. & Rizq, R. (Eds.) (2019). *The Industrialisation of Care. Counselling, Psychotherapy and the impact of IAPT* Monmouth, UK: PCCS Books.

Kousoulis, A.A. (2019). *Prevention and mental health: Understanding the evidence so that we can address the greatest health challenge of our times* London: Mental Health Foundation.

Kousoulis, A.A., Goldie, I. (2017) Mapping mental health priorities in London with real-world data. *The Lancet Psychiatry. 4(10):*e24.

Kousoulis, A.A., Goldie, I. (2018). The window of opportunity to improve mental health is now open. *BMJ, November.*

Layard, R. (2005). *The depression report: A new deal for depression and anxiety.* LSE: CEP.

McLeod, J., & Elliott, R. (2011). Systematic case study research: A practice-oriented introduction to building an evidence base for counselling and psychotherapy. *Counselling and Psychotherapy Research, 11:* (1–10).

McManus, S., Bebbington, P., Jenkins, R., & Brugha, T. (2016). *Mental health and wellbeing in England: Adult psychiatric morbidity survey 2014.* Leeds: NHS Digital.

NICE (2009). *Clinical Guideline 90 Depression in Adults.* London: BPS & Royal College Psychiatrists.

NICE (2011). *CG123. Common Mental Health Disorders. Identification and Pathways to Care.* London: BPS and Royal College Psychiatrists.

Pickett, K.E. & Wilkinson, R.G. (2010). Inequality: an underacknowledged source of mental illness and distress. *British Journal of Psychiatry 197(6):* (pp. 426–428).

Radden, J. & Varga, S. (2013). The Epistemological Value of Depression Memoirs: a Meta-Analysis. In K.W.M. Fulford, M. Davies, R.G.T. Gipps, G. Graham, J.Z. Sadler, G.

Stanghellini & T. Thornton (Eds.), *The Oxford Handbook of Philosophy and Psychiatry* (pp. 99–118). Oxford: OUP.

Rawlins, M. (2008). *De testimonio: on the evidence for decisions about the use of therapeutic interventions.* Lancet. Dec 20;372(9656):2152–61. doi: 10.1016/S0140–6736(08)61930-3.

Rose, N. (2019. Foreword. In Jackson, C. & Rizq, R. (Eds.). *The Industrialisation of Care. Counselling, Psychotherapy and the impact of IAPT* Monmouth, UK: PCCS Books (pp. v-x).

Solomon, A. (2001). *The Noonday Demon: An Anatomy of Depression.* London: Vintage.

Turpin, Clarke, Duffy & Hope (2009) A new workforce to deliver IAPT: a case study *The Journal of Mental Health Training, Education and Practice, 4(2),* 37–46.

Van Stolk et al (2014) *Psychological Wellbeing and Work: improving service provision and outcomes* RAND: Europe.

World Health Organisation (WHO) (2008). *The global burden of disease: 2004 update.* Geneva.

Index